But Hope is Longer

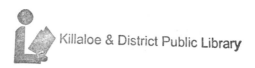
But Hope is Longer

Navigating the Country of Breast Cancer

TAMARA LEVINE

Second Story Press

Library and Archives Canada Cataloguing in Publication

Levine, R. Tamara
But hope is longer : navigating the country of breast cancer /
R. Tamara Levine.

Issued also in an electronic format.
ISBN 978-1-926920-89-4

1. Levine, R. Tamara—Health.
2. Breast—Cancer—Patients—Biography.
I. Title.

RC280.B8L48 2012   362.19699'4490092   C2012-904031-2

Editors: Sarah Swartz, Ruth Chernia
Designer: Melissa Kaita

Cover photo © iStockphoto

Printed and bound in Canada

*Second Story Press gratefully acknowledges the support of the
Ontario Arts Council and the Canada Council for the Arts for our
publishing program. We acknowledge the financial support of the
Government of Canada through the Canada Book Fund.*

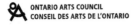

MIX
Paper from
responsible sources
FSC® C004071

Published by
SECOND STORY PRESS
20 Maud Street, Suite 401
Toronto, ON M5V 2M5
www.secondstorypress.ca

To my parents,
Helen Zivian Levine and Gil Levine

CONTENTS

Introduction

I was in the throes of despair when I wrote the first of my "Dear friends and family" letters on August 26, 2009, a few weeks after being diagnosed with Stage III breast cancer. I'd had a clear mammogram ten months before finding the lump. How could my healthy and resilient body have suddenly become so sick?

I struggled to get my head around believing I had cancer as I groped my way through the cancer care system. Discouraged and frustrated, I kept hitting the wall as I tried to come up with a treatment plan that made sense for me. Whatever the plan turned out to be, I knew I'd have to brace myself for the assault that cancer treatment would imminently inflict on my body.

I also had to face the possibility that I might not make it. What about my family? What would having a sick mother/daughter/wife do to my young adult kids? To my husband? To my elderly parents? What would it be like to be sick at home full-time after decades in the workforce?

My first letter was a way to let my world know what was happening to me, to get back to the people from various parts of my life who had phoned, e-mailed, and sent cards, flowers, and food since hearing my news. In that letter I wrote about fearing "both the cancer and the horrors of the treatment that await me." While I couldn't have articulated it at the time, I was also preparing to immerse myself in what I would come to call the "paradoxes of cancer."

The responses to my first letter were overwhelming. I hadn't imagined that some recipients would in turn pass my letter on to others, so I was bowled over by how far and wide it soon traveled. The messages that flowed in expressed shock and outrage, love and solidarity. They helped quell some of my fears about being left behind or forgotten as I prepared to drop out of my life as I had known it. While I felt more alone than I had ever been, it gave me some measure of comfort to know there were people out there rooting for me. What astonished me wasn't just the warmth expressed and the support offered, but how my letter seemed to have touched people's lives. The responses, as well as what was becoming my own burgeoning need to write, convinced me to carry on with the letters.

I had written on the job and penned letters, poems, and new lyrics to old tunes all my life, but now, for the first time, my writing was becoming intensely personal. There was no so-called objectivity or distance from what I was living at any given moment. I discovered that when I wrote from inside my experience, the letters resonated with readers in unexpected ways. I also came to realize that the writing itself was a kind of therapy – that it could transport me to a place of healing like almost nothing else.

I carried on with what I came to call my Healing Journey letters over the next sixteen months. I wrote through feeling rotten and less rotten, through fear, vulnerability, infirmity, visual impairment, despair, and hope. The letters became much more than a way to share news of what was happening to me. They became, in effect, "my work."

My letters became a chronicle of my seeing things in new ways. In the first letter, I wrote about feeling as though I had "entered a country which no one wants to visit, where a language is spoken that is vaguely familiar yet distant until now." I didn't know then that Susan Sontag had written about the idea of dual citizenship in her essay "Illness as Metaphor" in 1977:

> Illness is the night-side of life, a more onerous citizenship. Everyone who is born holds dual citizenship, in the kingdom of the well and the kingdom of the sick. Although we all prefer to use only the good passport, sooner or later each of us is obliged, at least for a spell, to identify ourselves as citizens of that other place.

The idea of being transported to a new country, of being an unwilling (and unwitting) immigrant or even a deportee became a recurring theme. Although we are surrounded by people who are going through, have been through, or have been lost to cancer and we hear about it regularly, it was completely different when cancer struck *me*. In an instant I was uprooted from all that was familiar and dropped into a strange, inhospitable, and dangerous land. The language of the new country had words with a familiar ring: tumor, malignancy, carcinogen, metastasis, chemotherapy. While I had a cursory, even detached notion of these words, each term took on a dreaded new and deeper meaning when it suddenly applied to my body and my life.

Once I had crossed the border from the land of the healthy into this new country, I couldn't help but notice the faces, bodies, and dress of its inhabitants. The scene was shocking to me, not because I hadn't seen people with cancer before, but because now they/we were gathered together as a collectivity, even a culture in the anthropological sense. As I looked around me, I wondered: are these "my people" now?

I was already marked, of course, but not yet visibly so. In those early days, I could still "pass" as a tourist and even return incognito to the world of the seemingly healthy. I still had my hair. My skin still had decent color, I had good energy and was feeling limber. But I knew it wouldn't be long before I would cross over and take on the pallor, dress, and gait of this new place.

Soon after my diagnosis, I went on sick leave and later on long-term disability. My work had been rewarding, intense, and demanding. Leaving it because of cancer was difficult: who would finish the course I was writing? Who would I be without my work-defined identity? What would happen to my relationships with colleagues and work-connected friends across the country? How would I now spend my time?

Almost overnight, my job became to get well. It was nothing short of a full-time job to get to all the appointments for tests and treatments. I spent vast amounts of time just waiting in doctors' offices and hospital waiting rooms, where I came to understand the meaning of "patient" in new ways. When I wasn't feeling horrible, I also saw my job as trying to keep my body as strong as possible. In a modified way, I tried to carry on with my fitness routines when I could.

Throughout treatment and beyond, with some serious bumps along the way, I was fortunate to have doctors who were not only at the top of their science but who were also warm, caring, and compassionate human beings. The "team" came together in part because of luck and circumstance. But it was also because of my efforts to be "captain of my own ship," as I was determined to find the best practitioners I could within both mainstream and complementary medicine. I was grateful to be able to form relationships with each of them over time that allowed us to explore aspects of life that went beyond regular check-ups and consultations.

After my first couple of Healing Journey letters, I began to sign off with "Be well. Carpe diem." It was the first time I had used *Carpe diem* as a closing salutation, but it soon became the trademark way to end my letters, notes, and messages. Carpe diem, Latin for "seize the day," summed up where I was at, and pretty much said it all in two short, powerful words from antiquity. When my mortality was on the line, the future was murky and unpredictable at best. It meant that all I could count on was *now*, and *now* in turn took on a whole new meaning.

Carpe diem fit well both with my newfound headspace and with the high drama my body was going through. If I was solidly grounded in the present, I was newly able to experience each day as it arrived. Not knowing how much time I had left or what tomorrow would bring, I could treasure each day, each relationship, and each experience as a precious opportunity. Even during my most wretched days, I'd try to find a glimmer, a ray of light and hope to hold on to. I'd choose what made my heart sing.

Margie Wolfe, a friend and the publisher at Second Story Press, had been receiving my letters from the beginning. She encouraged me to expand them into a deeper story about my cancer experience that would resonate with others and become a resource of broader interest. As I finished treatment and began to feel better, I started to write in earnest, digging deep into the recesses of my memory to fill in the stories behind and surrounding the letters. It was different to write from the vantage point of looking backward rather than from inside the experience. What the newer writing lacked in immediacy, it hopefully gained in insight as I peeled off the layers of my cancer journey and reflected on what I had learned. Sometimes, it was difficult to find the discipline to write, because there was so much else I wanted to do with my newfound health and growing energy. But the writing also drew me in. It became an increasingly powerful way to process my experience and come out the other side.

Along the way, I decided to interview my healers: Dr. Shailendra Verma, my medical oncologist; Dr. Joanne Meng, my radiation oncologist; Dr. Leesa Kirchner, my naturopathic oncologist; and Dr. Angel Arnaout, my surgeon; meeting with each of them in their office, in their home, or in mine. With their permission and with the tape recorder running, I asked them why they do this work, how they see breast cancer, what works well within the system, and what needs to change. I asked about their views on integrating mainstream and complementary medicine and about what keeps them going in the face of loss. I also interviewed Joyce Hardman, my life coach, about how she supports her clients who are going through breast cancer. The wise voices of these healers are woven into the story and into the last chapter of this book.

Folk music has always been an important part of my life. When it was time to come up with a title for this book, I remembered the lyrics Pete Seeger had added many years ago to the haunting spiritual "Jacob's Ladder." In one of the verses, he wrote: "Struggle's long, but hope is longer / Brothers, sisters, all." I've always loved the song and that verse because it not only recognizes the struggles and hardships of life but also shines a light of hope into darkness. "But hope is longer" summed up how I saw my travels in the country of breast cancer.

While this story is about my journey through and beyond breast cancer, my hope is that it will inspire others who are dealing with other cancers or other catastrophic illnesses. Whether you are a patient, survivor, family member, friend, health practitioner, caregiver, or whether you simply want to learn more about the journey, I hope you find something useful, meaningful, and helpful in *But Hope is Longer*.

Be well. Carpe diem.
Love, Tamara

CHAPTER ONE

The Nightmare Descends:
Getting the Diagnosis

It happened in the shower after an early morning walk with my friend Denise. It was mid-June and the dawn air had been fresh and cool, misty over the canal. Rivulets of soapy water cascaded down my awakened skin, and I felt grateful to start my workday with air, exercise, and good conversation.

As the water beat down and I lifted my arms above my head to soap up my underarms, my fingers slowed to hover as they came upon a strange round bump in the hollow of my left armpit. I thought back over my recent physical exertions, wondering what it could be, a pulled muscle maybe? Had I pushed or pulled too hard in one of my workouts? Had something sinister happened when I'd had my underarms waxed recently? As I prodded and probed the alien protrusion, I felt no pain or discomfort, just the smooth contours of a lump the size of a walnut that seemed to have sprung from nowhere.

I dressed and went downstairs to the kitchen, got my coffee,

7

grapefruit, cereal. My husband, Larry – eight years older than I am, now a woodturner in retirement – was already at the table, absorbed in the newspaper, eating, drinking his coffee, his gray, pony-tailed head bowed.

"Hey hon, guess what. There's a lump in my armpit. I found it in the shower, it popped out of nowhere."

He put down the paper, looked up, wrinkled his nose, and donned his glasses. With my arms raised up, he got up and stood behind me, his hands easily finding the lump. I'd been thinking I'd give it a week to see if it would go away, but when Larry said "Why don't you get it checked out?" it seemed to make sense. Thus began the whirlwind of appointments, scans, tests, waiting, and more waiting.

First I saw my family doctor, who examined me and found not only the lump in my armpit, but another lump lurking in my left breast. I took a deep breath as I watched his brow knit, steeling myself as he uttered the words *breast* and *cancer* in the same sentence, his face markedly concerned. It slowly dawned on me that the lump in my underarm might be in my lymph nodes and that it could be connected to the lump in my breast.

Is that how it happens? Did this mean that if I had cancer, it had already traveled from my breast to my lymph nodes? Why hadn't I been more vigilant about examining my breasts? Could I have found it sooner?

"Of course, there's a chance it's a benign cyst," said the doctor, "but you'll have to go through the tests to find out for sure." His nurse made an appointment for a mammogram.

What was happening to me? I was fifty-eight years old and had always thought of myself as healthy and resilient. I exercised, ate well, felt pretty good and had plenty of energy most of the time. I'd had yearly mammograms since turning fifty and the last one, ten months before, had been clear. I was at a good point in my life. I'd experienced the joys and battle scars of mothering, step-mothering, and a long marriage. The kids – Eric (age thirty-six), Rachel (age twenty-six), and Daniel (age twenty-three) – seemed to be at least semi-launched. I had a good relationship with my parents, who were living in the same city as I, and in relatively good health. I had a warm circle of women friends. I had worked all of my adult life, for the past twenty years as a literacy co-ordinator and adult educator in the labor movement. Larry and I had recently returned from a work trip and holiday in New Zealand, where I'd been invited to work with staff and to deliver the keynote speech for the NZ unions as they prepared to launch their new workplace learning program.

But if I had cancer, everything would change. I tried not to race ahead of myself as I made the rounds through the battery of tests over the next five weeks: a mammogram, two ultrasounds, and an MRI. I was frustrated with how long it was taking, doing my best to carry on with my life in a wary haze through the steamy days of July. At work, I tried to focus on the new course on conflict resolution I was writing to be piloted at the end of the summer. But as each test led to another that would explore further what was going on in my body, the possibility of cancer loomed larger. The final test involved having biopsies taken at the Women's Breast Health Centre, a hub of services within the Ottawa Hospital dedicated to all aspects of women's breast health. There, needles drew samples of tissue from my breast and underarm to be tested in the lab. The results would be available in a week or two.

Larry and I had plans to go to the Blue Skies Folk Festival a few days after the biopsies. This had become a beloved family tradition over the last twenty years, and we planned our summer vacations around it. I called my doctor's office to say that I'd be out of town for four days over the long weekend in case the biopsy results came in while we were away. I wanted to hear about the results as soon as they became available.

Now grown, the kids hadn't come to Blue Skies for several years, so it had become an adult venture. That summer, we were camping with our friend Cathy and her sister. Though there had been attempts to simplify packing over the years, the house was still piled high with camping equipment, duffle bags, sleeping gear, boxes and coolers filled with food, and my guitar ready to load. I was glad to be preoccupied with getting the food together, organizing and packing, since the familiar rhythms helped cut through the terror that was stalking me. I took a deep breath as we drove off that morning, relieved that the sky was clear. It looked like there would be dry ground for setting up camp, and we hoped our favorite well-worn patch of ground at the top of the hill would be waiting for us.

We arrived at the site, in awe of how the rolling fields had been transformed once again into the perfect setting for a folk festival. We carted the gear up to our coveted spot, set up the tent, and unpacked mats and sleeping bags. We hung a rope clothesline between two trees, put up the kitchen tent with its fly for shade and shelter and found places for food, water, dishes, and basins.

Being at Blue Skies seemed familiar and ordinary, yet remarkable and poignant at the same time. I wondered whether I'd be well enough to make it to another Blue Skies – or whether I'd even be alive this time next year. I wondered about the fears that must be lurking in Larry's head, Larry who had lost his mother to breast cancer when he was twelve and she thirty-five after going through the barbarous treatment of the 1950s.

I didn't feel much like socializing, but it felt safe to be in our small circle on the hilltop. Cathy and her sister were both keenly aware that the threat of cancer was weighing heavily on our minds. Cathy had gone through an aggressive breast cancer eight years earlier, and her sister had been her devoted caregiver then. So thoughts of cancer were there for all of us, hovering like a storm cloud over our conversations and silences.

On the first evening, the air was unusually balmy as we nestled in low chairs listening to the music. Communication with the outside world was difficult from Blue Skies. We had planned to take a break that evening to use a borrowed cell phone to call for news about a job interview our daughter, Rachel, had had that day in Montreal. As the stars began to appear in the night sky, we reached her from a spot that had some possibility of reception. Rachel asked over the crackling line, "Mom, are you in a quiet place?"

GETTING THE "NEWS"

I knew it then, before she had a chance to say it. The results had come in to my doctor's office earlier that day, and he had called and left a message on our voice mail. Our son, Daniel, alone at home, had picked up the message that said I had been diagnosed with breast cancer. With no way to reach us at Blue Skies, he had called Rachel, my parents in Ottawa, and my sister in Toronto. My whole family knew about my diagnosis before I did. I hadn't expected to get the biopsy results till the following week, but now I was hearing the news knowing Daniel had received it alone, and that my family had been dealing with it for hours.

Larry and I walked back slowly to the hilltop, leaning into each other, collapsing into the folding chairs under the fly of the kitchen tent. With my arms crossed tightly across my chest, I tried to understand how my kind family doctor of several years could have left the dreaded message on our voice mail. Had he simply been trying to let me know as soon as he could? How could this be happening when I had had a clear mammogram last summer? Had I done something wrong?

The nightmare that hangs over every woman's head had befallen me. I had three friends and a few acquaintances who had been through breast cancer, including one still in treatment and another in palliative care, but this still felt like an invasion from an alien place.

I wondered: am I going to die from this disease? Why don't I feel sick? How will I cope when my body is assaulted and mutilated by treatment? There was still so much we didn't know. What did the biopsy report say? How aggressive was my cancer? What was my prognosis? What would happen next? Also, who am I now that I have cancer? How can I just drop out of my life to deal with this?

I thought about my breasts, how I had been both excited and embarrassed at their precocious development. My first bra. Their erotic history over the decades, the pleasure they had given and received. My bittersweet experience with their primal nurturing function, my rage at pornographic depictions of breasts, especially right after I had given birth. The hard time I'd had after my kids were born trying to nurse each voracious baby, my "little barracudas," as the nurses called them. I eventually settled into nursing and loved it, grateful we all had persevered.

For the most part, my breasts had served me well throughout my life, but I had never before had to question their very existence, their longevity, the prospect of their violent demise. Wouldn't they always be part of me? Had they outlived their usefulness? What would it be like to have a body with only one breast? No breasts? Had my breasts betrayed me? Had I betrayed them?

Nerves frayed, raw, and exhausted, Larry and I crawled into the tent early that night. I slept fitfully, shifting around, restless, searching for a comfortable position in the sleeping bag. Lying in the darkness, I sought out each lump, now a full-fledged tumor, first in my breast and then in my underarm, caressing them as my fingers traveled back and forth like a tongue seeking a chipped tooth.

We got up the next morning and drove to the pay phone at the gas station on the highway. With the smell of gasoline in the air and cars whizzing by, I cupped my hand over my ear as I strained to hear the voice of each kid, my mom, my dad, and my sister. My voice broke as I stumbled through the conversations, fear palpable at both ends of the line, each trying to reassure the other. It was good to make the connections; to know my family was solidly planted in

Montreal, Ottawa, and Toronto; and to hold onto each other across the wires.

We went back to the festival, staying on to do our shifts in the kitchen. Soon I was chopping mounds of cherry tomatoes, green onions, and olives for the salads we would be putting out to sell a couple of hours later, glad to be preoccupied by such routine tasks. I shared nothing of my cancer; it was still too new, raw, private. I knew I wasn't ready to put the quivering, bloody mess of my news on the table, to make it available for view or comment, however sympathetic those around me might be.

We ended up staying at Blue Skies for the rest of the weekend. It was a good place to be – free of demands, expectations, or the phone – where we could safely move between listening to the music, hanging around the campsite, talking or silence. In the end, it was a welcome hiatus between getting the diagnosis and facing the world.

Cathy listened through the weekend, sharing stories and insights that had emerged from her own cancer experience. She offered understated suggestions, nuggets in the rough I wouldn't fully appreciate until weeks or even months later. "You'll have to be captain of your own ship," she said, referring to the need to be proactive when confronting the lack of co-ordination within the cancer care system, "because no one else will do it for you." I would remember her words on many occasions to come.

I had a hard time believing her when she said, "This won't make any sense now, but there will be gifts that come out of this." All I could think was, *What fucking gifts?*

Arriving home meant the usual unpacking, loads of laundry, and the "best shower of the year." It also meant that we had to begin dealing with the outside world and the cancer care system. That night, I started to make calls to friends and family who had been waiting for the test results. Often, there were tears at the other end of the line and I would end up sobbing too, drained after each call in spite of the support that flowed my way. In time, I gave the job of contacting others to a small group of my closest "connectors" – Larry, my mother, my sister, and two friends.

The next morning, friends Teresa and Tom arrived at our doorstep bearing flowers and pastries. Having each been through their own experience with cancer years before, they had received my phone message and knew instinctively to head over. Sitting around the dining room table, Larry and I shared our worries with them about the kids getting the doctor's message first. A father of three, Tom's words brought some degree of comfort, putting the situation in a new light when he said, "You know, it's unfortunate in lots of ways, but maybe it's not so terrible that this time the kids had to figure out how to take care of you."

Before we hugged good-bye, Teresa lifted up her summery top and bra to show me the faded pink lines that ran under her arm and across her breast, triumphant battle scars from her lumpectomy and lymph node dissection of several years before.

FIRST STEPS

Later that afternoon, my family doctor gave Larry and me a copy of the biopsy report. The mostly unintelligible fine print indicated that my "infiltrating ductal carcinoma" had "an infiltrative proliferation of epithelial cells surrounded by desmoplasia," "a high nuclear grade," and "tumor necrosis." Other than confirming that the cancer had spread to my lymph nodes, he wasn't able to explain what the details of the report meant or what my prognosis might be. We talked about what would happen next: He would make an appointment for me with a surgeon at the Women's Breast Health Centre who would recommend the kind of surgery I should have and set a date for it. I would see an oncologist after the pathology report from surgery became available when a plan for further treatment would be put into place.

With an appointment with the surgeon set for a week hence, I moved between feverishly getting the necessary things done and finding myself immobilized. Finally, the day arrived, and Larry and I were ushered into an office by a warm, capable nurse to meet the surgeon, a large white-haired man in his sixties. He, too, was

Dr. Joanne Meng: Family doctors generally refer their newly diagnosed breast cancer patients to surgeons as the first point of entry into the cancer system. But family doctors have very limited training in oncology with little or no specific training in dealing with breast cancer. There are few with the knowledge and skills to even talk about cancer with their patients.

unable (or unwilling) to tell me about the nature of my cancer from the biopsy reports, saying that the results so far were not conclusive enough and that a prognosis could only come following surgery. At that point, he would discuss the pathology report and I would be referred to an oncologist for further treatment. He told us he had more than twenty-five years of experience doing breast cancer surgery, announcing that he would perform a "partial mastectomy" on me. When he said he would preserve as much of my breast as he could, he looked across the room at Larry.

I asked whether we should consider doing chemotherapy before surgery. His reply was no, that it would not be appropriate in my case. He did not explain why. I also asked about seeing an oncologist before the surgery. I said I wanted to see Dr. Shailendra Verma, an oncologist I knew of by reputation through my breast cancer survivor friends, as soon as I could. Almost dismissively, he said I could but that it would not be useful, as the oncologist would need the pathology results that would only be available post-surgery.

Larry and I looked at each other in dismay when he said the wait time for my surgery would be at least six weeks. When I expressed concern about the dangers of a long wait time and its impact on the progress of my cancer, the surgeon replied that the delay would make no difference.

I became increasingly uneasy when I asked what he thought about the idea of exploring complementary therapies such as naturopathy and acupuncture. He told me not to waste my money, that there were lots of quacks out there trying to make a buck off desperate people.

The whole experience with the surgeon didn't feel right to me. Although he may have been technically competent, I found him patronizing and sexist. His secretary called a couple of days later to give me a surgery date more than seven weeks away, apologizing for the delay because it was summer, with doctors and other staff on vacation. It was already almost two months since I had found the lump, and another seven weeks would take my wait time to well beyond three months. Since the cancer had already spread to my lymph nodes, where else might it be traveling? My cancer wasn't on vacation; it had already been rampaging through my body for at least the last few months. I wondered whether I should consider going to another city with shorter wait times.

> Dr. Joanne Meng: Education and training are key. We need to build in communication and sensitivity training throughout medical school. We need better training for the surgeons who have a hard time understanding the whole picture.

AN INDIVIDUALIZED TREATMENT PLAN

Looking for support and trying to distract myself from my fears, I headed to a lunch date that had been organized by my "survivor sisters," friends who had experienced breast cancer themselves. We spent three hours at an Italian restaurant talking about coping with our diagnoses, finding our way through the cancer care system, trying to stay sane. Along with the stories, suggestions, and offers of practical support, I was grateful to have these women in my life. They had been through it and had come out the other side, and they understood at a visceral level what I was going through. But as I got up to leave, I suddenly felt dizzy, hot, and weak and knew I had to get home fast.

I was in bed within an hour, overcome by waves of fever, weakness, and a searing pain in my underarm. When I woke the next morning, still gripped by fever and pulsating pain, I knew I needed help. But there was nowhere to turn, as both my family doctor and the surgeon were on holidays. The only person I could think of calling was the nurse I had met at the appointment with the surgeon. When I told her what was happening, she suggested I go to a walk-in clinic to get a prescription for drugs to treat the infection. She also promised to call Dr. Verma, the oncologist I had hoped to see, to try to get me in to see him quickly.

I had no idea what to expect at the clinic. Thankfully, the doctor on duty that Saturday morning had lots of experience with cancer. When I showed her my inflamed underarm and the biopsy report, she could tell me that the high nuclear grade indicated that my breast cancer was highly aggressive. She also said the infection was probably related to the cancer in my lymph nodes and prescribed heavy-duty antibiotics. She expressed grave concern about the wait time for surgery, telling me about one of her patients who went to Toronto for breast cancer surgery where the wait time was shorter. She wondered whether I should receive chemotherapy first. She assured me I would be in good hands with Dr. Verma, whom I was to see three days later.

When Dr. Verma's secretary called before my appointment to say he was sorry he couldn't spend the usual length of time with me because they'd squeezed me in, I knew there was something special about this man besides his stellar reputation as an oncologist. Larry and I weren't sure what to expect as we waited in his examining room armed with our list of questions when a tall, flamboyant, silver-haired man in his fifties with sparkling eyes and a huge smile strode into the room.

Dr. Verma greeted us and gave me a hug before asking me how I was doing. He sat down in front of me with his knees touching mine, looking straight into my eyes. "You've been through a lot," he said as my tears welled up. As his practiced hands deftly palpated my tumors and the breast tissue surrounding them as I lay on the examining table, he confirmed that my infection was cancer-related and that my cancer was aggressive. I had a tumor of 2.5 cm in my left breast and one in my left axilla (underarm) that had increased from 5 to 8 cm with the infection. The cancer was a Stage III on a scale of I to IV because it had spread to my lymph nodes and was thus considered to be "locally advanced." It was Grade 3 on an aggressivity scale of 1 to 3. He said I would probably need a mastectomy, but that it would be up to the surgeon.

I was taken aback when he asked if I was Ashkenazi (Jewish of Eastern European origin), surprised that a doctor of East Indian background had readily eyeballed my ethnicity. "I'm recommending you go for genetic counseling to see about getting tested," he said matter of factly. I knew about the higher incidence of genetically based breast cancer in Ashkenazi women, and thought immediately of my daughter. I asked if the testing would be for Rachel's sake and was surprised when he said no. It would be to help determine the type of surgery I would need.

"If you have the gene, we'd probably recommend a double mastectomy and removing your ovaries to try to avoid the cancer coming back in the other breast or ovaries. The rate of recurrence for women with the mutated gene is higher," he said. "But we've got some time because we're not going to do surgery first. We're going to attack your cancer systemically, not locally. We'll do chemo first, eight rounds instead of the usual six. You'll come every three weeks starting as soon as possible, probably within a few days. We'll make sure you get the drugs you need to get through the side effects."

Dr. Shailendra Verma: We apply chemotherapy to women with more aggressive, locally advanced cancers because the outlook is more grim with a greater chance of a relapse. If it's more serious from the get-go, why not look at it systemically from the outset?

Finally, I had landed in good hands. It struck me that my wretched underarm infection had been a blessing in disguise because it had got me on the right track. It was a complete fluke, but I now had an oncologist who had made a wise judgment call to fit my individual circumstances. Taking a systemic approach made so much more sense than putting me under the knife first. Even though there was lots of scary stuff in what Dr. Verma had said – the aggressivity of the cancer and treatment, the prospect of a mastectomy or worse, what might show up in genetic testing – I was relieved to finally be on a more solid path with a treatment plan based on my individual diagnosis. As the first few rays of light started to filter into the black hole, I thought about Cathy's advice to be the "captain of my own ship."

My meeting with Dr. Verma and the decision to start treatment with chemo meant that my seven weeks of waiting had shrunk to a mere seven days. Rather than having what seemed like an abundant, albeit nerve-wracking, amount of time to get my head and body together for surgery, I now had just a week to do everything that needed to be done.

There had been many calls and missives as people far and wide from various parts of my life, past and present, work-related and personal had phoned, e-mailed, sent and brought over cards, flowers, gifts, and food. Often, I hadn't been able to return the calls or thank people directly for their thoughtfulness. Before chemo started, I wanted to write to thank them and let them know what was happening with me.

I also wanted to tell the people who still hadn't heard my news. I wrote my first group e-mail letter on August 26, 2009, to about fifty family members, friends, and colleagues. It was the first letter of what would become my Healing Journey.

✉ Healing Journey #1

August 26, 2009

Dear friends and family,

This is a hard message to write, but I wanted to let you know that I have been diagnosed with breast cancer. I have been in touch with many of you personally, but know that there are some of you with whom I haven't had the chance to connect. I found it difficult and upsetting to make the first calls, and after a few tries, decided to ask a few "connectors" to get in touch with others. My deep apologies to those of you I was not able to reach before now.

After finding a lump in my underarm toward the end of June, I saw my family doctor who found a second lump in my breast. My mammogram ten months earlier had been clear. A mammogram, an ultrasound, an MRI, and a biopsy followed over the next month or so, culminating in the diagnosis of invasive ductal carcinoma (ductal because it originated in the duct, invasive because it had spread to my lymph nodes). The cancer appears to be aggressive. But there is still much we don't know, like how far it has spread and what the prognosis is.

Until yesterday, the plan had been to undergo surgery on September 30th, a frustrating 3+ months after finding the lump. But after an inflammation in my underarm developed a few days ago with swelling, fever, weakness, and pain, I was able to see an oncologist yesterday. (It seems that typically, oncologists aren't usually in the picture till after surgery, when they determine the next steps in treatment based on the pathology of the tumor tissue that has been removed.) My oncologist is recommending a "systemic approach," which means starting me on chemotherapy next week for twenty-four weeks, followed by surgery.

Needless to say, the news has been devastating for me, my

family, and friends. The nightmare that hangs over every woman's head has descended upon me, and everything changes, all plans, priorities, preoccupations. I have always thought of myself as healthy and resilient, but now I fear both the ravages of cancer and the horrors of treatment that await me. I have shed more tears than I can ever remember. I feel that I have entered a country which no one wants to visit, where a language is spoken that is vaguely familiar yet distant until now.

At the same time, there have been blessings. The support of my family, the outpouring of love from my friends, the insights of my women friends who have survived this scourge, and the offers of help from so many of you have done wonders to support me and bolster my spirits as I prepare for the fight of my life. I am on sick leave, as my job now is to get as strong, healthy, and centered as possible in the days leading up to treatment.

I'll try to keep you posted on next steps as the saga unfolds. If I don't respond to your messages right away, please know that I appreciate them and will respond when I can.

Love,
Tamara

Reflections

EVERY WOMAN'S NIGHTMARE: GETTING A CANCER DIAGNOSIS
Every woman who has been through breast cancer has a story to tell about how she received her diagnosis. During the long weeks and sometimes months leading up to it, each of us is painfully aware of how the cards appear to be increasingly stacked against us. As one test result begets another and then another, we know in our hearts that the conclusion is likely to be cancer. Yet we hope against hope that it will be otherwise: that the lump will turn out to be a benign cyst or that there will be an error in one of the tests.

As much as we psyche ourselves up and brace ourselves for what seems to be inevitable, we are never prepared to hear the news "You have breast cancer." But of course we need to know, and so where, how, and who we are with when the message is delivered is of paramount importance. Here are some essential ingredients:

- The diagnosis should be given or received in person, never over the phone. If a message is left, it should ask the patient to call the doctor's office for an appointment as soon as possible.

- The patient shouldn't be alone when she receives the diagnosis. She should be encouraged to bring a trusted family member or friend to the appointment who will serve as her advocate and note taker. This person must not take over or speak for the patient: she or he needs to respect that the appointment is for the patient who is primary in the encounter. The job of the friend or family member is to provide support and take thorough, legible notes for future reference.

- The news needs to be delivered by a doctor who understands the biopsy results and who can explain them to the patient with compassion, accuracy, and clarity. If the patient's family doctor cannot do this, the patient should immediately be referred to a specialist who can.

- The appointment must be long enough for the doctor to tell the patient what her diagnosis is and to explain what it means, and for the patient to react to the news and to ask questions. The doctor needs to respond with understanding and with clear and accessible answers. There should plenty of time for emotions to be expressed and responded to.

- The doctor should give the patient as much of an idea as possible of what the next steps will be. This includes the time frame for treatment, the potential ramifications of the various treatments, and how the patient will be involved and kept informed of choices and decisions regarding her treatment now and along the way.

- The patient has to know who to contact about the questions and concerns she will have following this appointment. She also needs to understand the role of her family doctor during her treatment.

"I HAVE BAD NEWS": HOW TO TELL THE WORLD?

It was hard enough to hear the news of the diagnosis, to absorb and process it, let alone think about how to tell the world about it. Breast cancer is "more than a disease." It affected not only my health but also my identity and my sexuality. The diagnosis represents a seismic shift in our sense of ourselves, of who we are, and what our lives will be from now on. No matter what our particular diagnosis entails, we face the loss of ourselves, our health, and our place in our families and in the world.

As so many of the underpinnings of our lives disintegrate before our eyes, we ask ourselves, "Who am I now that I have breast cancer?" We brace ourselves as we

Dr. Angel Arnaout: All the things that traditionally were never measured are now starting to be more important. It has been shown that your cancer outcome improves if you feel better about yourself.

contemplate facing treatment and anticipate the pain, disfigurement, and un-wellness it will bring. We can hardly imagine what it will mean to reconcile ourselves to the chance we may not survive.

If it's like that for us, how do we tell the rest of our world? How do we put into words what we need to say to our spouses, children, parents, and siblings? How do we tell our friends? What do we say to our employers and co-workers? There are no easy answers, and so much will depend on the nature of the relationships involved.

I wanted to be as emotionally honest as possible with the people closest to me. I wanted to say less about the litany of facts associated with my cancer than about how I was experiencing the wretched diagnosis. I needed to remind myself that it was up to me what I chose to share and with whom.

"I have some bad news. I've been diagnosed with breast cancer. I know I'll be going through surgery, chemo, and radiation, but I don't know a lot more than that." We can be that brief and to the point, without going into a lot of detail. It's okay for us to say we don't know the answers to particular questions, because there will always be lots of unknowns.

The writing and sending out of my first Healing Journey letter was an important way to let people know what was going on. While others offered to send messages, I knew I wanted the news to come from me. I didn't want my story to be filtered through anyone else's lens. The writing was an important step for me in starting to take charge of my situation, to become the captain of my own ship in my own words. It also meant I would receive the responses, which arrived like embraces from across the miles.

AWKWARD MOMENTS: THE RESPONSES

There is no doubt that most people we encounter as we run the gauntlet following diagnosis are honest and well-intentioned. They want to wish us well, but they sometimes struggle to come up with what they consider appropriate things to say. They end up trying too hard, and what comes out doesn't ring true and isn't helpful.

As a newly diagnosed breast cancer patient, the exhortations to "think positively" were among the hardest to take. I found myself bristling when well-meaning acquaintances and co-workers urged me to be "positive." I wanted to say "I can't think positively when I'm in despair. I've just received the worst news of my life. I need you to respect where I'm at. If you tell me that thinking positively will influence my outcome, you're dismissing what I need to be doing right now. But if you respect how I'm feeling, I'm more likely to feel your support and come out the other side. Once I've worked through my grief, I hope to be stronger, more determined, and ready to fight this cancer because of it."

I felt let down when a couple of friends I thought would be there for me didn't come through. I also had a hard time with a few people who went "technical" on me, who wanted to know the "facts" without clueing in to my emotional state. It felt as though they were more interested in the data about my cancer than they were in me, although they may well have been trying to shield both of us from the rawness of their real emotions.

I also had trouble with "How are you?" Mostly an innocuous greeting with an honest reply rarely expected, it threw me every time, even when it came from strangers. When the friendly cashier at the supermarket asked me "How are you?" I found I was struck dumb, seized by the dilemma of whether I could lie or withhold the truth in my reply. It was liberating to realize that I didn't have to tell her or anyone else my whole story; that it was all right to take a deep breath and say, "Okay, thanks." I fared better if people simply empathized, looked me in the eye, said "Oh shit" and gave me a big hug.

This doesn't help:

- Asking too many questions

- Making comments like "Think positively, it's all about your attitude" or "Everything will be fine."

- Pumping for "technical" information about what is going on

- Telling the story about your aunt, mother, sister, friend, etc., and her experience with breast cancer

This helps:

- Clueing in to my emotional state

- Looking me straight in the eye

- Allowing for lots of time and spaces of silence

- Not worrying about saying "the right thing": it's okay if you show emotion or don't have the right words.

GETTING ON TRACK IN THE HEALTH CARE SYSTEM

I was relieved to finally have a plan for my treatment that made sense. Dr. Verma's strategy to attack my cancer systemically with eight rounds of chemotherapy would start almost immediately. Once chemo was finished, I'd have a few weeks to recover before surgery, although I didn't know yet what that would involve. A month or so after surgery, the pathology report would indicate whether they had got all the cancer. This would be followed by twenty-five radiation treatments to irradiate any remaining cancer cells and help prevent a recurrence. If all went well, the whole process would take about a year.

It still disturbs me that I "accidentally" got on the right track for treatment. I wonder what would have happened if my particular circumstances had been different and I hadn't had some luck on my side. What if I hadn't got the infection in my underarm? What if I hadn't encountered the special nurse in the surgeon's office, and if she hadn't gone above and beyond her duties to get me in to see Dr. Verma so quickly? What if Dr. Verma hadn't been both a great doctor and a caring human being?

If I'd waited an interminable seven weeks for surgery, plus another month to heal and wait for my pathology, followed by another couple of weeks of waiting before starting chemotherapy, it would have been a total of five months since finding my lump. We know that women don't die from breast cancer itself but from how it metastasizes, or spreads, to other parts of our bodies, such as our lungs, liver, and brain. If I'd had to wait five months, who knows where my cancer might have traveled and what dire outcome might have awaited me?

There were so many questions: (1) Why is surgery assumed to be the first line of attack in every case of breast cancer? Is this practice a relic of the old-style radical mastectomies when the only recourse was to gouge out the tumor? If surgery is by definition a local intervention, wouldn't it make sense to start with a systemic intervention like chemotherapy when we know the cancer has already spread? (2) Why isn't each breast cancer patient looked at individually? (3) Why wasn't an oncologist involved from the beginning immediately following diagnosis? (4) Why wasn't a team of specialists (medical oncologist, radiation oncologist, surgeon, pathologist, radiologist, etc.) who would be involved in my case assembled right after diagnosis?

Dr. Joanne Meng: Radical mastectomies started to be done about 100 years ago. The problem was that they often didn't work, and the patient still died of breast cancer. The primary oncological premise is to remove the cancer first.

Dr. Shailendra Verma: It took a lot of dying women to convince the world that surgery was not the cure for breast cancer. We figured we had to come up with a more systemic approach to treatment. We always have to ask: if the treatment doesn't work, what should we do to make it work? The goal has to be less disfigurement and less suffering.

Shouldn't they meet to discuss what approach to take in my individual situation? If so, how and when would it all happen?

It all felt fragmented – a beleaguered system crying out for co-ordination. As time went on and I moved through the various way stations of cancer treatment, I would continue to ask questions and imagine what a better system might look like.

> **Dr. Shailendra Verma:** There's this elegance of an evolution in how we treat cancer. We've moved from excising cancer by the knife to systemically treating it with poison to a more sophisticated approach that says "One woman, one cancer, one treatment." We're not quite there yet, but it's the dream.

CAPTAIN OF YOUR OWN SHIP

As I began treatment, I remembered Cathy's words: "You'll have to be captain of your own ship." What does this mean? It means being proactive when confronting the lack of co-ordination in the cancer care system. It means you need to work hard to be resilient, strategic, and hell-bent on survival. You'll need to be curious, to inform yourself, to learn the new language, and to figure out how the medical system works in the country of cancer. You'll need family and friends around you, but you'll also need to make connections with others who are new arrivals in the country too, because they will understand what you are going through in ways no one else can. You can also learn from the older "travelers" who came before you and have wisdom to share.

How do you rise to the role of "captain" when you're feeling so helpless?

A few thoughts:

- You have the right to despair when you learn you have cancer. Like grief, you need to let yourself sit inside it and not short change this process. If you can face your emotions; allow them to roil, stew, breathe, and run their course; you will have a better chance of coming to a place of strength and be better able to face what lies ahead.

- You know yourself and your body best. You know better than anyone else how you handle stress, illness, and drugs. You also know what will help you heal and thrive and who you want to have around you. Doctors have valuable knowledge, expertise, and experience, but if you say, "Yes, doctor" because you are intimidated or uninformed, you will remain a passive recipient of care.

- Be your own advocate within the cancer care system and recruit others to help and support you when needed. You need to read and to seek out the advice, suggestions, and recommendations of those who have been through cancer before you. Who are the best oncologists, the best surgeons? Whom should we avoid? You have the right to ask for a particular doctor, and although you may not succeed in getting who you want, you have the right to ask for a second opinion. Most importantly, you need to ask questions and not settle for answers, treatment, or providers of care that don't feel right to you. Always ask: What is the best treatment plan for me?

- Explore the supports in your community in addition to the services and treatment offered by the cancer care system. Practitioners of complementary health care, such as naturopaths, chiropractors, massage therapists, physiotherapists, and nutritionists, as well as programs that offer fitness, yoga, meditation, and so on can help you fight your cancer, lessen the negative side effects of treatment, bolster your immune system, and promote your healing. At the same time, be wary of treatments and therapies that have not been proven to be effective.

- Seek out kindred spirits – those within your circles of family and friends as well as new people who give you emotional and practical support. Friends whom you might have hoped would be there may not come through while others may surprise you. A wide range of formal and informal support groups offer opportunities to find people on similar physical and emotional journeys.

- While others can be an enormous support, we are ultimately alone on this journey. It will help if we can discover what nourishes and sustains us, how to be in our solitude, what will help us weather the storm we are living through. Some of us will choose music, writing, art, meditation, yoga, gardening, cooking, or being in nature as our therapy of choice. The important thing is finding out what works.

No matter what, there will be rough waters ahead. But if we can stay as solidly as possible in the captain's chair with a strong crew around us, we'll have our best hope for the crossing.

CHAPTER TWO

Navigating Uncharted Waters: Treatment Begins

I mapped out my eight rounds of chemotherapy on the calendar. For the first four rounds, I would receive a combination of two drugs, doxorubicin (Adriamycin) and cyclophosphamide (Cytoxan), commonly known as "AC." For the last four rounds, I would receive docetaxel (Taxotere), a powerful drug known to be particularly brutal. There would be three weeks between each round of chemo.

Chemo started on September 3, 2009, and my last round was to finish on January 28, 2010. But Dr. Verma assured me these dates would soon go by the wayside because chemo schedules never go according to plan. There would be times when I couldn't receive chemo on schedule because my white blood cell count would be too low, or I'd be fighting a cold or flu that would inevitably set in due to my chemo-weakened immune system.

In preparation for chemo, I had to have a peripherally inserted central catheter (PICC) line inserted into my upper right arm. The

PICC line provided a protected route for the chemo to travel safely into a large vein, thus avoiding the danger of it "killing my flesh" with its powerful toxicity. Getting the PICC line was a painless procedure, but when it was done there was a spidery mass of thin tubes dangling from my arm with loose netting around them. A home care nurse would come to flush my PICC line once a week throughout chemo.

I was horrified when the technician told me I couldn't get it wet. I wouldn't be able to swim and I could only take a shower if I wore a plastic sleeve over it. Swimming has always been important in my life: how was I going to get through this if I couldn't swim?

The fateful day arrived. As I approached the chemo room for my first infusion with Larry and my sister Karen at my side, it felt like we were entering a giant fish bowl. There were hospital beds set up around its periphery, with the feet of each occupant pointing toward the middle of the room. A group of reclining chairs created a kind of inner circle. Nurses bustled about the IV poles that were attached to about thirty patients of all ages, male and female, some alone, others with company. Some patients looked completely at home cozily ensconced under colorful quilts, surrounded by the iPods, snacks, and teddy bears they had brought with them. Some looked relatively healthy, while others were pale and decidedly unwell.

The chemo room looked chaotic to me. It was hard to imagine how the nurses could keep track of which patients were to get which of the bags hanging from the ubiquitous poles. When a nurse set me up in a reclining chair in an alcove off the main circle, I guessed I was in the area reserved for new patients.

The first nurse checked my name and birth date to make sure she had the right patient. Then she asked whether I had a PICC or a "port." When I asked what a port was, she said a "porto-cath" is a small medical appliance surgically inserted beneath the skin of the chest. Connected by catheter to a vein, it is an alternative to the PICC line for receiving chemo safely.

A woman in one of the chairs nearby overheard us, and promptly pulled down the neckline of her top to show me a small, grape-sized bump in her chest. "It's great," she said, "and you only have to have it flushed at the hospital once a month. You can even swim with it. But it's minor surgery, so you'll have to go on a waiting list."

Why hadn't I known about ports before? Why hadn't I been offered one? Apparently, they had given me the PICC line because I'd started chemo on short notice, but also because it involved a cheaper, less invasive procedure. Aside from the encumbrance and inconvenience of a PICC line, I knew I had to find a way to swim if I was going to stay sane and survive chemo. I resolved to do everything in my power to get a port.

✉ Healing Journey #2

September 16, 2009

Dear friends and family,

First of all, a huge thank-you. The outpouring of love and support in response to my first "Healing Journey" message has been both bountiful and humbling. I have received heaps of flowers, e-mails, cards, gifts, and calls with your wishes for courage and hope. From near and far, you have shared your shock and outrage at the news, your generous offers of emotional and practical support, your stories of struggles with breast cancer. Most of all, you have sent your love. You have said you would pray, meditate, chant, and run races for me, and generally send your good vibes. It's all so overwhelming and powerful, so much appreciated.

Where to begin? So much has happened since I wrote to you as I was beginning my journey with breast cancer. When it looked like the first step in my treatment would be to have surgery on September 30th, I thought I would have seven weeks to prepare. My plan had been to spend the time getting as strong, healthy, and centered as I could. I would eat well, get lots of exercise and fresh air, and start to put the pieces in place at home and elsewhere that would help me get through treatment in the best way possible. In the end, when the direction changed completely after meeting my oncologist, I had just seven days before starting chemotherapy on September 3rd. It would be the first of eight rounds I would get every three weeks for the next twenty-four weeks, to be followed by surgery and radiation.

Those seven days were a whirlwind. One of the first things I had to deal with was my hair, as I knew it would start to fall out a couple of weeks after chemo began. My hair, which I had hated for its wildness until my thirties when I finally grew to appreciate and even love it, is part of who I am. It's my signature, my identity. Who would I be without it? How would it feel to be bald? Would I be brave enough to go bald outside the house? Would I have the courage to hang out bald with my friends, or swim at the Y? Should I get a wig? What about losing the hair on all the other parts of me?

The advice I got from my survivor sisters was to deal with my hair in two steps: first, get it cut short so the falling clumps wouldn't be so huge and upsetting; then have my head shaved to get rid of the wisps and patches once the falling was underway. So when my daughter, Rachel, arrived from Montreal to spend her two-week vacation in Ottawa with Larry, Daniel, and me, we took on the hair project together.

First we went to see Bruce, who had been cutting our family's hair for twenty-five years, from the time Rachel and Daniel were so little they had to sit on a board that straddled the arms of his big chair. When we told him about my cancer and about the kind of cut I was looking for, there were hugs and tears and we set up an appointment for a few days later. Then with Rachel and Louise, my friend and survivor sister who had been through her own journey with cancer, chemo, and hair loss, I went wig shopping at Freda's. There, a young hairdresser patiently helped me try on at least a dozen wigs in various shades of "silver." We even had some moments of hilarity when I tried on a curly white wig that made me look like the Queen, and I got to do my "Philip and I and the corgies" number before we settled on two wigs to put aside until I returned with less hair.

I have decided to pursue the complementary therapy route to supplement what I will be getting from my medical doctors. In addition to my wonderful massage therapist, chiropractor, and life coach, I found Dr. Leesa Kirchner, a naturopathic oncologist with extensive training and credentials in treating cancer and whose practice focuses exclusively on cancer patients. With the support of Dr. Verma, my medical oncologist, Leesa has put me on a regimen of supplements that both fight the cancer and help lessen the negative effects of chemo. She also gives me acupuncture treatments before and after each round of chemo.

Larry and the kids have embarked on a "tech" shopping project, as we decided that this was the time to finally give in to cell phones and an iPod, and that a TV and DVD player in the bedroom would help during the rough days ahead. Good-humored tutorials with the kids helped diminish my techno-peasant angst about learning to operate the gizmos (yikes)!

Rachel and I also went to my office to pick up a few personal things and to say *au revoir* to my co-workers at the Canadian Labour Congress. They had baked a cake and bought flowers, giving me hugs that morning that were especially big and warm with lots of good wishes for my health. I know I will miss them, but I'm also working hard on letting go, at least for now.

Larry and I had a good couple of days with the kids at the cottage just before chemo started. It was great to have time to just hang out together, to yak, play games, and have my last swim of the year in the lake. Driving home out the dirt road, we gasped in wonder as we came upon a black bear and her two small cubs, something we hadn't seen in our thirty years there. Completely awed by the bear family, its symbolism didn't hit me till the next morning when I bolted upright in bed with an overwhelmingly powerful sense that I was the mother bear and that I had to find a way to stick around for my "cubs."

When my seven days were almost over, Karen arrived from Toronto. We hadn't seen each other for a month, but we had talked on the phone every day since my diagnosis, and she had been an enormous support all the way along. She came with Larry and me to my first chemo session at the hospital.

It began with nurse giving us a barrage of information about side effects and a fistful of prescriptions for an arsenal of anti-nausea drugs. The first chemo nurse set me up on a drip, referring to the red liquid chemo drug that was flowing into me as the "red devil." When a second nurse came to detach me about an hour later, I asked if that was the end of the red devil. She said she didn't call it that, but called it instead the "red angel" because it was healing me. I was struck by the paradox: how can I learn to receive chemo and the treatments that will follow not as a terrible infliction on my body, but as a formidable and positive force that will heal me?

The five days following chemo are a blur of queasiness and lethargy. I had no appetite and the smell and thought of food repulsed me. My family tried to get small amounts of bland food into me, like tofu with scrambled eggs. They ran out to buy ginger ale and organized my supplements into charts and containers so that I wasn't totally overwhelmed. It wasn't as horrible as my worst nightmare, but I felt pretty lousy. At the same time, I tried to fight it, going for walks when I had a bit of energy in the mornings, going to pick up my wig, going out for a family supper on Rachel's birthday, trying hard not to give in to the full extent of my depletion. But it was a losing battle, and by the fourth day I started to come to terms with the fact that I had to stop planning, lie low, and listen to my body. Even if it meant lying down five times a day, that was what I needed to do. I seemed to manage a bit better after that.

On the sixth day after chemo, I pretty much got myself back. The queasiness and the exhaustion departed, and I had new energy and a bit more interest in food. Today is day fourteen, and I'm doing okay. I've had some good visits with friends and even got to the cottage on the weekend. They say that the post-chemo pattern tends to repeat itself with each cycle, although it's also cumulative so the tiredness will intensify. I'm watching how this cycle plays out in the hope that I'll have some good days next time too.

It's still early days. This is just the beginning. There is still so much I don't know about my cancer and about what awaits me, but we welcomed the news yesterday that the tests I had last week showed that the cancer hasn't spread beyond my lymph nodes and that my tumors have already started to shrink with the chemo.

I hate that this cancer has invaded me, and fear where it might travel. I dread the treatments that await me. I'm upset that this is happening to my eighty-five-year-old parents, to Larry, to my kids, and to my sister. And yet, at the same time, I can feel the total despair that infused the weeks following my diagnosis diminishing to some extent. I've noticed that my tears flow less abundantly and less often, and that I'm gripped less frequently by the terror of what lies ahead. I don't get as thrown by the question "How are you?"

I wonder if I'm moving to a new stage of this living with cancer, although I'm not sure what it is yet. After wandering in the desert for the first month after the diagnosis, I feel confident about the team that is in place for my care now: Dr. Verma, my medical oncologist, my radiation oncologist, and surgeon as well as Leesa, my naturopathic doctor. I think I'm finally on the best possible track for treatment.

I'm working hard to accept what is positive within "the paradox." Even my hair falling out will mean that the chemo is working because it's attacking my rapidly growing cells! I'm appreciating the "special glasses" I seem to be wearing these days, a kind of heightened awareness that lets me see people and the world in new ways. I'm drinking up the amazing love and support that so many of you are sending my way.

Once again, I hope you will forgive me if I'm not always able to get back to you individually when you write or call. I'll do my best to keep you posted on my progress. Thank you again for being there in so many wonderful ways.

Love,
Tamara

Reflections

FAMILY SUPPORT

The seven weeks that became the seven days I'd have to prepare for treatment felt like a genesis, my own version of the creation myth that would require enormous upheavals in the universe in abbreviated amounts of time. While I was relieved to be starting treatment right away, the imminent start date was a major shift from the time I thought I'd have to gradually collect myself; take care of practical matters; organize my surroundings; and get as healthy as I could.

The support of my family made getting through these daunting tasks possible, as they put much of their own lives and preoccupations on hold to help out. Rachel spent most of her badly needed holiday coming with me to say good-bye at my office, see the naturopath, get my hair cut, and go wig shopping. Larry and Daniel went shopping for a new TV, DVD player, and portable sound system for the bedroom and set them up. Daniel figured out a system for the array of naturopathic supplements I'd started to take, organizing them into a chart and putting them in a container with color-coded troughs for each day of the week. Rachel and Larry came with me to the information session on chemo at the hospital. My parents checked in with me every day, offering to help, visiting often, and distracting me with games of Upwords, a favorite family word game. My sister came from Toronto for my first round of chemo and spent the first post-chemo weekend with me, vowing to come in for each post-chemo weekend to follow.

I worried terribly about my elderly parents, fearing what my illness might do to them. I thought: *Let nothing happen to my parents as I go through cancer and treatment.* They were both still feisty and engaged with the world, but at the same time they were also increasingly frail, grappling with old age, losing friends, and facing their own mortality. They had watched closely as I went through the battery of tests and received the diagnosis, baffled at how all of this could be happening to their once strong and healthy daughter. It was hard enough for them to cope with their own realities without having to anticipate the possible death of one of their children. Losing a child of any age defies the natural order of things, turning everything upside down. They rallied valiantly to my side, anxious to support me in every way they could.

Like all families, mine is a complex organism. Each person has particular strengths: some were able to be there completely on an emotional level, while others were better at helping in more practical ways. Inevitably, there were moments of both disappointment and triumph. I worried about how everyone was doing and what kind of support we'd need to get through this time.

I was concerned about Larry, who had lost his mother to breast cancer. What it would be like for him to relive those emotions with me so many years later? As we sat on our back deck one afternoon in the waning September sun I asked, "What are *you* going to do to get through this?" He said that although there would be rough times ahead, he was managing under the circumstances, and if he needed to talk, he'd speak to a friend. I worried that he'd need more than that if we were going to make it. I wondered whether we should be going for family therapy.

There were growing pains involved with the new configurations on the home front. Being home based for the first time since my maternity leaves decades ago was a major switch, as the house had been Larry's exclusive daytime domain since he'd retired years before. After honing his skills as a woodturner, he now produced exquisite bowls and platters out of his basement workshop. With me home full-time now, I wondered if he'd feel that his space had been invaded.

Larry gamely picked up much of the work around the house. He wanted to know how I was feeling and what I needed, and always came with me to my medical appointments. He spent most of the rest of his time in his workshop, checking on me during the course of the day if he knew I was feeling crummy. Sometimes that was okay, but at other times I felt alone and bereft, wishing he'd stay with me even if there wasn't anything practical to do. I wondered what he was thinking about, what his fears were, where he was really at. I knew Larry loved me and that he was scared, but his minimalist responses to my questions told me it was sometimes too hard for him to go there.

In the evenings, depending on how I was doing, one of us would make supper. Then we'd eat and talk about what was happening. Afterwards, we'd sit at the dining room table and play Upwords, listen to music, and drink pots of green tea, each of us craving, amid the chaos, a semblance of normalcy in our time-worn rituals.

Reluctantly, Larry fielded many of the calls and offers to visit me or bring food over, taking on the task of gatekeeper. He believed he was trying to protect me from too much activity and minimize the toll he feared the visits would take, but I often felt he was overly zealous in the role. I worried that his rigorous gatekeeping wasn't only for my benefit, but that it was likely also serving his own increasingly reclusive inclinations.

Because it wasn't how he would have done it, Larry had trouble understanding how much I needed and depended on the support of my friends. I stressed that my friends were an essential part of helping me get through this time, pointing out that he didn't have to be part of the visits if he didn't want to be there. I know there were lots of times when I went overboard, when I should have stayed quiet, declined a visit, or insisted on a shorter one. The fine balance between how much, how little, or how often I, or we, had people over would remain a source of tension between us over the coming year.

There are no easy answers for dealing with family dynamics when the mother/wife/daughter/sister is going through breast cancer. It is a time of unprecedented fear and stress for everyone, when solidarity within the family is needed more than ever. In the best possible scenario, the foundations of the family relationships are already solid and there is a history of being there for each other on which to build.

The patient will be weaker and more fragile because of everything that's happening to her. Her family may tiptoe around her, wary of asking questions or afraid to talk about their fears in order not to upset her. This is a time when the patient needs to be clear and forthright about what she needs from her family, both practically and emotionally. She can set the tone by being as open as possible about what she is thinking and feeling and encourage others to do the same in an age-appropriate way. Everyone will benefit from a spirit of generosity and lots of hugs.

Often, it is the patient who has been "the strong one" in the family, the emotional rudder, the connector, the one who co-ordinates and takes charge. While it can be an upheaval when her multiple roles appear to be coming undone, it can also be an opportunity for others to move in. Sometimes, her new vulnerability can invite more openness and a taking on of new roles and tasks by others.

I had been seeing Joyce, my life coach, for about a year when I was diagnosed. I was grateful to have her as an important support in my life again after a gap of many years, especially since I knew she had coached several women through breast cancer.

It is worthwhile to consider getting professional help for members of the family, including the patient, either individually, as a family, or both. Finding the right counsellor is key, because a good therapist can be an important sounding board, troubleshooter, and support during a difficult time. It is a sign of strength, not weakness, to seek help in times of crisis.

TOO MUCH INFORMATION?
There were so many questions about cancer and I needed answers. I picked up a couple of books and started reading, beginning with the

breast cancer "bible," *Dr. Susan Love's Breast Book*. Larry spent hours reading it. I flipped through its pages, searching the index, scanning paragraphs and pages here and there. The book helped ground us with solid information about breast cancer and about what to expect from treatment. But in my perusing, I'd also come upon bits of ominous text that might apply to my situation and I'd catch my breath and close my eyes in a vain attempt to shield myself from the dreaded "facts" as I tried to contain my fear.

It is a blessing and a curse that there is so much information about breast cancer available. It's everywhere: at the hospital, in doctors' offices, and in libraries and bookstores, and of course on the Internet. But how do you know what information will be useful at any given time? What if you find contradictory information? How much of it can you absorb? How much will you be able to handle emotionally? Is there such a thing as finding out too much?

I hesitated about the Internet, knowing how overwhelming and terrifying it could be. But there were times when its allure was too powerful, when I couldn't help myself and I'd go there anyway, bracing myself as I read furtively until I got scared. Then I'd turn off the computer and walk away.

The Internet can be a frightening place, one we can enter surreptitiously at any time of the day or night. It can be seductive, even mesmerizing, with tentacles into an infinite number of sources of information that range from sketchy to trustworthy. When I went there in my times of sheer terror to find out where my cancer might take me, it was usually against my own better judgment.

I went, for example, to learn more about what it meant that my cancer was "locally advanced" and what the five-year survival rates were for women with breast cancers like mine. Each time, after surfing around for an hour or so, I'd end up slamming down the laptop as if it was Pandora's box because I had discovered something newly terrifying.

There were also times when information I found on the Internet was useful and practical, like when I needed to find out more about the impact and side effects of a particular chemo drug.

If you go to the Internet, it is important that the sites be reputable and up to date, with accurate and clear information. Start with major cancer organizations, hospitals, and recognizable support groups, and networks. If you're so inclined, there are also hundreds of blogs and chat lines available where women who are in our shoes ask and answer a whole gamut of questions, tell their stories, and provide testimonials.

Sometimes, it's easier to ask others to search the Internet. Friends and family are often looking for ways to be useful and are pleased to do something concrete and practical to help. They will likely have a more dispassionate eye when searching for information that the patient may find especially loaded, and they can use their filters to sift out the essentials before transmitting the information.

THE BEST OF BOTH WORLDS:
CHOOSING COMPLEMENTARY CANCER CARE

I knew little about complementary cancer care when I was first diagnosed. But when my mother handed me the name and number of a naturopathic doctor who worked with cancer patients, I was curious. I knew naturopaths had a holistic approach to healing and that they used a variety of strategies, including nutrition and natural supplements, to support the immune system and strengthen the body's ability to heal itself. But could they help with a disease as catastrophic as cancer?

I soon learned the difference between alternative and complementary (or integrative) cancer care. The goal of complementary care is to work with mainstream oncology with the purpose of complementing, enhancing, and ideally integrating with it. Alternative care, on the other hand, is an approach to health that is usually practiced independently or outside of mainstream health care.

I had always been open to alternative approaches in my life. I read as much as I could about complementary approaches to fighting cancer that are used in tandem with conventional treatment. I read about the value of naturopathy, diet, supplements, vitamins, acupuncture, and other therapies. Once I had Dr. Verma looking after me and a solid treatment plan in place, I trusted that I'd be in good hands within the cancer care system. But at the same time, the idea of straddling mainstream and complementary medicine made sense to me. I wanted to find out if naturopathy could complement the treatment I'd be getting from the cancer center. If I was going to do everything possible to fight my cancer and be as healthy as possible through treatment, I wanted to take advantage of the best each had to offer.

I made an appointment to see Dr. Leesa Kirchner before I started chemo. I felt fortunate to find out about this naturopathic oncologist who works exclusively with cancer patients and survivors. I wanted to start working with her early in my cancer treatment so that it would indeed be complementary. At our first meeting, I found her to be knowledgeable and compassionate. She invited me to call her Leesa. Together, we came up with a plan to fight the cancer, lessen the side effects of chemo, and build up my immune system. I started on a range of supplements and made plans to see her for acupuncture before and after each round of chemo.

Although I now had a stellar medical oncologist, it didn't necessarily follow that he would know about or be receptive to looking at what naturopathic oncology had to offer. Leesa told me of examples in other countries

Dr. Leesa Kirchner: When you're going through conventional treatment, naturopathic care can help mitigate side effects. Therapies that are studied and proven can help patients finish treatment by diminishing side effects. Quality of life is paramount. It can prevent neuropathy in a patient. Or it can mean a patient who has been given two months can go to a birthday party and feel okay.

where naturopathic doctors work alongside medical doctors in cancer clinics and hospitals, often supported by the public health care system. In Canada however, using a naturopath during cancer treatment is still unusual and considered "offbeat." She lamented the lack of knowledge of naturopathic medicine by many Canadian oncologists and other cancer specialists. She warned me that her patients sometimes encountered problems when their doctors weren't familiar with what naturopaths do and thus didn't support their intention to work with her. Some doctors scared their patients into thinking that seeking naturopathic care would undermine the benefits of their cancer treatment, advising them against it or even forbidding them to get involved. I had run into this kind of disparaging attitude from the first surgeon I had met.

LEAVING WORK BEHIND

Although it was no longer foremost on my mind, I knew I needed to deal with my work life. I had to tell my employer what was happening, and find out about what was involved in taking sick leave and getting long-term disability. I had also recently been elected as chair of the board of directors of Inter Pares, the social justice organization to which I was deeply committed as a volunteer. I would have to let the staff there know what was happening so we could figure out a back-up plan. I needed to reorganize my life to fit with my new reality.

My doctor had told me I would probably be off work for at least a year. Ironically, I had only become a permanent employee in the education department of the Canadian Labour Congress a couple of years earlier after being a temporary workplace literacy co-ordinator in two organizations for almost twenty years. Along with a permanent job, I had been presented with my long-term disability (LTD) card. Before tucking it away in my desk drawer, I remembered taking a long look at it, fingering it, feeling grateful for it, and hoping I would never have to use it. Yet for the first time, here I was about to start three months of sick leave followed by LTD, which would cover about 70 percent of my salary. I thought of the women with breast cancer who didn't have such benefits or even sick leave, about what it would be like to be worrying about making ends meet on top of everything else they were coping with.

When I first learned of my diagnosis, I was scheduled to pilot a new course I was in the process of writing. I was anxious that it be ready as part of our labor education school taking place at the end of the summer. In the blur of receiving the news about my cancer, I found myself still thinking about the course: what I had to do to get it ready, whether there was a chance I could be there for the pilot. Based on my assumption that I'd have surgery first, I calculated the timing, thinking my surgery probably wouldn't happen until September, after the course. Afterward, we could find someone to write the revisions and carry out the next steps. Reeling from the news of my diagnosis at the same time as my head was swimming with the details about the course, I was still seeing it as "my baby."

Thankfully, it was Cathy, my friend, colleague, and survivor sister whose wisdom prevailed. "You're not going to be able to be at the school," she said gently. "You'll be going through a whirlwind over the next few weeks. You'll have all kinds of medical appointments to go to, and that's before you even know what your treatment plan will be. You'll have a ton of details to take care of in your own life." It was a stroke of luck that Cathy, also a union educator, was signed on as a co-facilitator for the course. "Don't worry about the course. You've laid the groundwork," she said. "We'll figure it out." I knew in my heart of hearts that Cathy was right. It was clear I'd have to let go, but what did that mean?

I'd been working full-time for more than thirty-five years, essentially all my adult life. I loved the popular education work I was doing, especially when I was facilitating groups of workers who arrived in my classes from every imaginable kind of workplace. I'd had the opportunity to do education work in many parts of Canada. While my work environment was often demanding, the job was a good fit with my commitment to literacy, feminism, and social justice, and my love of writing and learning. Although I felt I also had a rich life outside of work, there was no question that my work was central, and that it gave shape, meaning, and context to my life.

It wasn't that I couldn't imagine the idea of not working or that I had difficulty being away from work. Although I often worked intensely and for long hours, I wasn't a workaholic. I was able to relax and enjoy life, and I savored my down time. I had been thinking that I'd probably work three or four more years before contemplating the idea of retirement.

But what was happening to me now had nothing to do with choosing. This was different: my cancer was precipitous, unexpected, and unplanned. When I searched for language to describe how I was feeling, *catapulted* came to mind. It was as if I had been suddenly catapulted into an altered state of being by a calamitous force of nature.

I had to find a way to make sense of the diagnosis alongside the grim truth that I'd have to separate from the work that was so much a part of my life and identity. What would it be like to close the door and walk away from it all? Who was I if I had to leave my work-identified self behind? What would happen to the friendships and the other important relationships that were so intimately connected to my work? What would the fabric of my days look like now? Would I ever be able to go back?

I felt like a snake having to shed its old skin. Unlike the snake, which sheds its old skin as it outgrows and literally busts out of it, I was shedding several layers of skin simultaneously. I mourned each layer of myself as I imagined it loosening and separating from me before I sloughed it off and watched it fall to the ground: my resilient good health, my identity, my hopes for a vibrant future. The shedding of each successive layer of skin left me even more naked, raw, and vulnerable. At that point, I had no sense that there was any regeneration underway or that there would be anything to replace the parts of myself I was losing.

It was all I could do to take on what had now become my new "job" of getting on track with my treatment plan, fighting my cancer, and getting well. Cathy was right: as soon as I left Blue Skies, the whirlwind began. My days filled up with tests and medical appointments as well as visits to my naturopath, coach, massage therapist, and chiropractor. I made sure to get exercise every day and tried to eat well. I started to write the Healing Journey letters. In the end, it was a relief that my work responsibilities were taken up by others. It meant I could focus my time and energy on getting well.

Some women decide to keep on working full- or part-time through treatment, usually out of necessity but sometimes out of choice. Some find ways to continue to work, but take time away from their regular routines to accommodate their treatment schedules and "black-out" days when they are too tired or sick to work.

Women continue to work for a wide variety of reasons:

- out of financial necessity

- because they have run out of sick leave and lack support from their employers to take additional time off

- because they are self-employed

- because working feels like a better choice, allowing them to maintain some normalcy and routine in their lives, or because it keeps them busy, allowing them to focus on something other than their breast cancer.

I wonder too, whether there are some women who keep working because they want to believe they can do it all or because they are in some level of denial about having breast cancer. *If I'm still going to work, can I really be sick?*

There is also all the unpaid work of women that is "never done:" the childcare, cooking, shopping, cleaning, laundry, gardening, yard work, chauffeuring, and so on that all women do to greater or lesser extents. In most households, we do most of the emotional and care-taking work too. Sometimes, there is help forthcoming from our spouses, children, or paid services. But what happens to all that work when we get sick? In my mind, the best thing is for (a) other family members to take over the essential work; (b) friends to help out with meals, errands, driving, etc.; and (c) everyone's expectations to be drastically lowered. The ideal situation is that women get the financial, practical, and emotional support we need and deserve in order to go through our treatment and focus on our health as successfully as possible.

A NEW WAY OF BEING: THE BODY RULES

I soon learned that my life would be irrevocably altered during chemo and that I would need to listen to my body. The director of my department, who had retired just before I was diagnosed, had invited the group who had planned her retirement party to the best restaurant in town to thank us. Planned weeks before we knew what my treatment schedule would be, it turned out that the dinner would be taking place two days after my first round of chemo. It had never occurred to me that I might not be able to attend.

I had gone for acupuncture treatments with Leesa before and after my first round of chemo, I was on an assortment of naturopathic supplements, and I had taken my anti-nausea pills as the chemo nurses directed. I didn't feel horrible in the hours that followed chemo, but by the next day I felt queasy and lethargic. By mid-afternoon it became clear that the idea of going to the dinner was ridiculous. The strongly scented aromas of the rich food would be sure to further nauseate me, and I probably wouldn't last more than an hour at a gathering that would go late into the evening. With sadness, I called to say I wouldn't be able to make it.

The next day, Karen and I walked the few blocks from our house to the local farmers' market. It was a glorious September day, sunny and warm, with nature's bounty piled high on the fruit and vegetable stands, a rainbow of bold colors glistening in the sun. As we wandered through the market, poking around the crafts tables and buying apples, I held my breath as we passed the stands of fresh baked goods, trying not to gag at the overpowering scent.

We found a bench after fifteen minutes or so, my legs weak and rubbery from walking. As we sat there people-watching, a favorite activity we had learned at our mother's knee, I marveled at how strong and healthy everyone around us seemed to be, and how I, in contrast, was not. It was a strange new way of seeing the world. I realized that I needed to come to terms with this new way of being. I had always been able to count on my body, but I had to accept that I was now living on another plane. There was no point fighting the truth that my body had to rule, and that I had no choice but to go with its needs and demands, fickle and unpredictable as they might be. Plans from now on would have to be understood by all parties to be tentative, made with the proviso "to be confirmed." While it was a tough reversal from my familiar patterns and especially from my expectations of myself, it also gave me some relief as I reluctantly settled into my new reality.

It was still early days, but it seemed like a pattern was starting to emerge in my chemo cycle. I would manage for a day or so following treatment, then I'd feel rotten for three or four days. Afterward, the weakness, queasiness and lethargy would gradually start to lift, and by the end of the week, I was close to being myself again. There is no doubt that finding out the cancer hadn't spread beyond my lymph nodes and that my tumors were already shrinking from the chemo helped raise my spirits. I only hoped the pattern would continue so I could count on having two not-so-bad weeks out of three.

CHAPTER THREE

Letting Go: Traveling with Chemo

It was an adjustment, but I was starting to get used to living my life according to the three-week cycles of my chemo schedule. Before each treatment, I'd go for a blood test at the hospital lab to make sure my white blood cell count wasn't too low for me to receive chemo. Low white blood cell counts are common among cancer patients: while chemo is attacking cancer cells, it is also attacking your immune system and lowering your resistance, which means that colds, coughs, and other infections are more likely to set in. When this happens, treatment is delayed until you're well enough to receive it. If the cell count is good, you get the green light to go ahead with chemo.

I also saw Dr. Verma a couple of days before each round of chemo. Larry and I would sit down together the night before my appointment and think about the questions we wanted to ask. In a small examining room where I changed into a blue hospital gown, one of the nurses would weigh me and ask about the side effects I was experiencing. Then Dr. Verma would come in and greet us warmly, shaking our hands and often giving me a bear hug. He always asked me how I was doing before he examined me. As he palpated my left breast and underarm, I'd search his eyes and face for clues of what he was finding, then wait anxiously for the news.

I was relieved to hear that my tumors were already starting to shrink. Being able to "see" evidence of the chemo working is a major advantage of going through chemo before surgery, because the tumors are still in place and their shrinkage can be monitored. If the tumors aren't shrinking, the oncologist can explore the possibility of switching to a more effective chemo drug.

On the negative side, a further check of my biopsy tissue for the "markers" or characteristics that defined my particular cancer revealed it to be "triple negative." Aggressive and more difficult to treat, triple negative cancer isn't fuelled by estrogen or progesterone or by the HR-2 protein. With no hormonal therapy (such as tamoxifen or one of the aromatase inhibitors) currently available to help prevent a recurrence following treatment, there is a lower survival rate than with other forms of breast cancer.

Dr. Shailendra Verma: It was only a few years ago when we started to notice that women were responding differently to treatment based on the particular biology of their cancers, the markers which define them as estrogen, progesterone, or HR2 positive or negative, etc. We've taken one disease and made it into six or nine or twelve. These markers can help predict how the cancer will behave in the future and how it will respond to treatment. We've entered the era of trying to target the particular breast cancer to help women survive the disease.

With this news, I found myself drawn like a junkie to the Internet that night, surfing for information on triple negative breast cancer. I discovered 10 to 15 percent of women with breast cancer have the triple negative markers. When I learned that most of us are pre-menopausal and of Hispanic or African descent, I wondered how this scourge could have befallen me. The only positive news was that we can respond well to chemotherapy, especially when the cancer is discovered in its early stages. What I found confirmed that I was on the right path by doing chemo first. But when it also sent me into a quagmire of fresh despondency, I knew I had to find a way to "let go" of my fears and any semblance of control I was still holding on to.

Cancer has a way of putting things in perspective. Here was another paradox: at the same time as I was striving to be my own captain, I also had to accept that any control I thought I might have had over my life and my destiny was an illusion. Along with my work, my status in the world, my identity, my good health, my hair, and my plans for the future, I would need to relinquish all vestige of control.

✉ Healing Journey #3

October 14, 2009

Dear friends and family,

It feels like it's been ages since I last wrote to you. So much has happened over the past month. It is the best of times and the worst of times. Maybe that's just how it is these days.

The shape of my life has changed completely, and has come to revolve around my cycles of chemotherapy every three weeks. All together, I will have eight cycles of chemo, four each of two different drugs. So far, I have a crummy first week following treatment when I'm queasy and lethargic. These are my post-chemo "black-out" days, as I have come to call them. Thankfully, the crummy week in my first two cycles has been followed by two pretty good weeks when I am in good spirits with energy and an appetite. As I near the end of my second cycle, I'm grateful to be feeling well as I brace myself for what my third cycle beginning tomorrow will bring.

It's tough, but I'm making some progress in coming to terms with the "chemo paradox," as I try to receive the infusion as a source of healing rather than one that makes me sick. It helped to get the good news that the cancer hadn't spread and that the tumors were shrinking. There was more good news a couple of weeks ago when I met my new surgeon (her name is Angel!) who told me she would be able to do a lumpectomy instead of the mastectomy I was anticipating. It's been a struggle that included an impassioned letter to the Ottawa Hospital about problems I encountered in the "black hole" of the cancer care system, but I now have a "dream team" of medical and other practitioners in place. With the help of my coach, Joyce, I'm hoping to be able to accept my vulnerability and yield to the mystery of what lies ahead.

I decided to go ahead with my doctor's recommendation to have genetic testing for a mutation of my BRCA gene, which serves as a suppressor of breast tumors when healthy. If the tests indicate there is a mutation, however, there is a much higher risk of recurrence, which could mean more invasive surgery.

I've joined a breast cancer support group at the hospital. It's way too big – twenty-six of us ranging in age from thirties to seventies – but it's a sign of how many of us are going through this, and we're only the ones who can get there. It's still great to meet women who are also in the middle of breast cancer treatment, and where losing our hair and breasts or parts thereof becomes a new kind of normal. The stories, the sharing of wisdom and the support are invaluable.

I find myself reading the obits differently now. I've read them for years to see if I knew anyone and for interesting and quirky details about people's lives. Now I read them with a special interest in women of my generation – who they are, the shape of their lives. I look for the cause of their deaths, which is sometimes explicit and sometimes not, so I read between the lines. I don't think it's being morbid so much as being curious about the lives of women who have been where I now find myself.

With all the changes in my life, I am surprised that it has not been as difficult as I would have imagined to "let go," at least of some things. When I asked Kai, Cathy, and Adriane if they would take over responsibility for finalizing and delivering my course at the Canadian Labour Congress summer school, for example, they responded with compassion and generosity. Afterward, I was grateful to be able to revel in the stories about the success of the course without feeling badly about having missed out on it.

It was hard to tell the staff and board members at my beloved Inter Pares about what was happening with me, especially after just being elected chair of the board in April. After I offered to step down or work with a co-chair when I was able, I was thrilled when a fellow board member was willing to step up to the plate as co-chair while I wend my way through treatment. Not really letting go, but a way to step back as needed.

I was not nearly as successful in letting go of my hair. I was aware of how my hair defined me to others, of comments that it was "distinctive" or "dramatic." What I didn't know was how much my hair defined me to myself, how painful it would be to lose it, and how bereft I would be without it.

I held on to my hair for about two weeks following my first chemo treatment before it started to come out when I tugged, brushed or washed it. My scalp was red and sore, as if it was angry that my hair was being forced out of it by the chemo toxins. I dreaded my impending baldness, wondering who I would be to myself and others without hair. I told my parents that they were the only ones who would know me because I had been a bald baby! At my second chemo treatment, the nurse noted that most patients had already lost their hair by then. Knowing it was a losing battle to hold on, I made an appointment to have my head shaved a few days later when my best-ever sister Karen, who is spending my black-out weekends with me, would be here from Toronto.

Now, I'm trying to get used to my hairless self, still startling when I look in the mirror and see my scalp in all its nakedness. Nakedness... first, a state of innocence, later, a state we can choose with whom to share it. But I haven't chosen this nakedness; it has befallen and devastated me.

I was working out at the Y last week when a woman noticed my cap and the armband for my PICC line. She asked if I was on chemo and what kind of cancer I had. When I told her I had breast cancer, she said I was lucky because I had a good chance of beating it. She had pancreatic cancer and was dying. We bonded instantly. I hadn't thought of having breast cancer as being lucky in any way, but I can see where she's coming from.

I wore my wig for the first time when I went out for lunch last week. I felt like a bit of a fraud, maybe because the wig creates an illusion of having hair while the other headgear covers me with less pretence. After lunch, I went next door to the bookstore. I was unprepared when a young saleswoman I knew there complimented me on my new haircut!

There is no question that my life has changed hugely and dramatically. Cancer is wretched, and the treatment in some ways is worse. When my survivor sisters told me early on about the "gifts" that would also come, I thought they were out of their minds. Now, two and a half months into this journey, I'm getting an inkling of what they mean. The outpouring of love and support continues to surprise and comfort me. Between the horrors of my treatment, there is a sense of the spaciousness I have long craved, bringing with it the possibility for the reflection I yearn for. My intuition seems to be deepening. There is no distance, no erzatz "objectivity," just the poignancy of being completely inside whatever experience I find myself in. I have started a letter-writing correspondence with my mom and a dream class at a yoga center.

Larry, Rachel, Daniel, and I celebrated Thanksgiving at the cottage on the weekend before shutting it down for the winter. The weather forecast was miserable, mostly rain. But it ended up being gorgeous, with the autumn leaves at their peak, sunshine and blue skies, and earthy forest smells. When my dad joined us on Sunday, we talked about what we were thankful for. We thanked the farmers for growing and harvesting the fabulous food on the table. We were thankful that I was now on the right track with my health care. I expressed my gratitude for the incredible support they each continue to give me.

Thanks too, to you for all that you give me from near and far. I hope you understand that though I dearly wish I could, I am not able to respond to each of you individually.

Thanks to Debbie and Denise who will be in touch with some of you who live close by and who have generously offered to help in different ways. So much appreciated.

Until next time, Carpe diem.
Love, Tamara

Reflections

WORKING IT OUT

I had been going to the local YM/YWCA for decades, where I did a cardio routine, weights, and stretching, and I had started swimming a couple of years before. I loved how my early morning workouts helped calm whatever worries were plaguing me and gave me the energy I needed for my day.

After I was diagnosed, it was hard to get my head around what it meant to be "healthy" now. If I had cancer, hadn't my body betrayed me? What was the point of trying to be in shape if I was already gravely ill? Even if I wanted to keep up with my exercise routine, how could I do it if I was going to feel so wretched?

As much as I railed against the cancer that had invaded me, I knew I had to find a way to make peace with my body. My body and I were in this together. I needed to believe that the cancer was contained in one small part of it, and that the rest of my body was as healthy and strong as it had ever been. If I could figure out how to be partners with my body, we could work together to be as strong as possible to fight the cancer and reclaim "our" life.

I wasn't sure how to "do" the Y as a cancer patient. I was weakened and depleted, I had an awkward, cumbersome PICC line dangling from my arm that made showering difficult and swimming impossible, and I knew I would soon be completely bald. There would be many days when I wouldn't be well enough to do much of anything, but I wondered if I could manage to do some kind of modified program during the two less horrible weeks of my chemo cycle.

If it was going to happen, my fitness routines would have to change. I'd get to the gym or walk with Denise when I felt well enough. If I couldn't make it, I couldn't give myself a hard time. I'd lower the bar several notches: it was okay if my pace was slower and

I took breaks as needed. Shorter walks, less time on the machines, less rigorous stretching. Fewer laps in the pool were fine, once I had the portocath. I had to be satisfied that whatever I was able to do was "good enough."

After my hair fell out, I worried about what to wear on my head when I was working out. I wished I could be one of those women who are willing to go out into the world unabashedly bald, but I was self-conscious and not ready to be hairless in public. The scarves, hats, and bandanas I'd been collecting would be sure to get sweaty and fall off during exercise. Then one day, I picked up one of the cotton caps Larry wore to protect his scalp when he was woodworking. I realized that his snug, blue cotton beanie was just what I needed. At last, with a new "uniform" that felt reasonably secure, I headed off to the gym.

The women I saw at the Y weren't friends, but they had been familiar faces for a long time, and I often chatted hurriedly with the early morning regulars as we flew between the locker room and the showers. Now that I wasn't working, I no longer had to get there at 6 a.m. or race through my routine, so I encountered a mostly new mid-morning crowd. I found it difficult when people didn't recognize me, although at the same time I was relieved to be "incognito."

I noticed that the mid-morning women were likely to be more relaxed, slower-paced, and less pressed for time than the early morning crowd because they weren't rushing off to work. Some seemed to be curious and interested in me, taking a few extra minutes to talk and listen. Once I began to feel less awkward with my new look and garb, I found that if I felt safe enough, I was able to tell a few of the women that I was going through treatment for breast cancer. Usually, they would respond warmly. From then on, they would ask how I was and how my treatments were going with genuine interest, encouraging me to carry on with my exercise regimen.

My new exercise routine became more than a workout. As I walked or sweated it out on the elliptical trainer, the rowing machine, or eventually in the pool, it became another way to "let go" of my fear, anxiety, and pain. It was never easy, but it did wonders for my body and spirit.

It's no doubt easier to figure out how to carry on with exercise when you already have a fitness routine that you can modify during cancer treatment. But it's also never too late to start exercising in modest ways, like going for short walks. The best part is the pay-off: almost immediately, it makes you feel better physically. It quells or at least cushions your angst. If you can get at least some of your exercise outdoors, you also reap the benefits of being out in the fresh air.

Exercise supports and fuels the body in its fight against cancer. It puts you in the best possible position to receive treatment well, while resisting its toxicity. It provides fortification for what lies ahead. It is one of the most generous gifts of self-care you can give yourself.

CANCER RELATIVITY

When the woman at the Y with pancreatic cancer said I was the lucky one, I was surprised. I felt anything but lucky. I never imagined that having any kind of cancer could be "lucky" in any way, and I had only a vague notion of what the survival rates were of the different cancers. But as I moved more deeply into the world of cancer, I discovered that indeed there were "better" and worse kinds to have. It has to do with survival rates determined by research that has analyzed the statistics on the outcomes of the patients who came before us. As Cathy pointed out during my early days, we're not yet a statistic when we're diagnosed because it's too early for us to be included in the research. But eventually we too will become a statistic, part of the growing body of knowledge that attempts to predict the prognosis and the future of those who will follow.

I became conscious of the pecking order among the various cancers each of us were dealing with as I sat in hospital waiting rooms and in Leesa's clinic where I spent hundreds of hours with other cancer patients. For example, the statistics on five-year survival rates vary greatly: pancreatic: 5%, lung: 15%, esophageal: 16%, brain: 30%, ovarian: 43%, colon: 64%, breast: 89% (triple negative: 77%, me: 50 to 60%), prostate: 99%.

Could my Y acquaintance have been right when she said I was lucky? Several months later, I read her obituary in the newspaper. I thought about the odds, about how they had been stacked against her. But even though she had considered me "lucky," relatively speaking, I knew my odds weren't so hot either. In five years, only slightly more than half of us with breast cancer characteristics like mine would be alive and only 20 percent of us would be cancer-free. If I could let go of the dreaded statistics, maybe it would help me focus on doing what was in my power to get well.

FELLOW TRAVELERS: CANCER SUPPORT GROUP

At one of my early appointments, I was given a package with information about a support group for newly diagnosed breast cancer patients. Led by the social worker at the Women's Breast Health Centre, it would take place once a week for six weeks. I thought it would be worthwhile to meet some women who were in my situation, so I decided to check it out.

I arrived with some trepidation at the hospital lounge for the first meeting. There was a buzz of instant recognition once we began to congregate. For the first time since I'd been diagnosed, I found myself in a roomful of women who were living and breathing the same experience as I was. It was an amazing feeling: Even if we had nothing else in common, we already knew a lot about each other.

As an adult educator, I worried that twenty-six was too large for a group like this to work well with one facilitator. But there was a backlog of breast cancer patients from over the summer and hospital resources were limited. We had to make the best of it.

We talked in groups of two or three until we were invited to gather in a circle of comfortable chairs and couches. Then the social worker asked us to introduce ourselves. My interest was piqued: I wanted to know more, to hear everyone's story and to offer mine. But it soon became clear that the agenda was set with structured topics and resource people and only brief snatches of time and space for personal sharing. I wished we could spend more time in small groups hearing from the women there, the real "experts," and find ways for all our voices, even the quieter ones, to be heard.

In spite of the constraints, the warmth and the terror we all harbored emerged each time we met. We connected with each other, urgently trading stories and information during breaks and before, between, and after the sessions.

When the group began, there were only two of us who were already losing our hair because we'd started with chemo first. The other was a young mother of two small children. I wondered about the women with young children, their terror of dying before their kids were grown, their worry about how to explain what was going on when they were sick or losing their hair or breasts, how they would cope with caring for the kids when they were feeling horrible. I felt grateful that my children were grown.

Most of the other women had recently had surgery, usually mastectomies. Or they were about to have surgery, and their chemo would be starting after they had healed. We talked about our fears of losing our breasts, our hair, our identities and possibly our lives. We exchanged stories and strategies for coping on our own, or with husbands and partners, children of all ages, and financial worries and for dealing with better and worse doctors, the medical system, drugs, sickness, and infirmity.

Being part of this support group soon felt like I had come home. It was a place where we peeled off hats and wigs as soon as we arrived, where we felt comfortable, even liberated in our baldness, and where we could safely let go of all pretenses. Our conversations zeroed in on what mattered most. Sometimes, a woman would break down in tears because of a situation she was dealing with, and we would rally around her with support and suggestions. A few minutes later, we'd find ourselves laughing uproariously at an anecdote someone had shared. It was an oasis where none of us was a minority.

WORKING WITH A COACH

I first went to see a life coach in 2000, when I thought I was about to lose my job. While I didn't end up unemployed, Joyce was an enormous help as we worked together over a period of several months to figure out my priorities. When we finished working together, she gave me a stuffed turtle: I needed to slow down and remind myself to take naps.

I had gone back to see her in 2008, and was especially grateful to have her in my life again when I was diagnosed the following year as I knew she would have a great deal to offer me now. Although she had never been a cancer patient herself, Joyce had been Cathy's coach and had worked with several other breast cancer patients.

Coaching is different from traditional therapy. Therapy is based on a healing model that looks at the pain of the past and helps us make peace with it; coaching is based on a wellness model. It is a process of accompanying and supporting us to clarify our vision of what and how we want our life to be. It helps build our skills in dealing with the roadblocks that are in the way of getting there.

Soon after I was diagnosed, while I was still in despair, I booked a session with Joyce. It occurred to me that she might be able to help me work on preparing my mind and body to receive chemo. The question that was foremost on my mind before my first round of chemo was: How can I learn to receive chemo, not as an assault on my body, but as a positive force? When I asked Joyce if she could help me work through this contradiction, she suggested, "Try to open yourself up to the idea that the infusion running through your veins is carrying energy that will heal you. While it may make you feel sick, remember that it also means the chemo is penetrating every cell of your body. It's tackling your cancer and will make you well again." It was an image I struggled to hold on to each time I visited the chemo room, that the toxic fluids dripping into my veins were healing me.

Joyce also helped me find ways to live with the uncertainty of whether I would live or die, and later, with my fears about the cancer recurring. It was another way I had to learn to let go: if I believed I was doing all I could to get the best of what mainstream and complementary medicine had to offer and if I continued to do all I could do to heal myself by eating well and exercising, then I'd have to accept that everything possible was being done. "Your challenge," she said, "is to accept that the rest is a mystery."

> Joyce Hardman: My job is to see helplessness as an opportunity. I've seen it in my own life and with each person who has gone through breast cancer or other catastrophic illness. I've experienced it again and again. It's a breakthrough into trusting that there is something bigger that holds me, that loves me, that it's not just me trying to keep it all together. It's part of the mystery I can't predict.

WRITING AS THERAPY

My days no longer consisted of working, traveling around the country to deliver courses, going to the gym before dawn, seeing friends, preparing meals for myself and others. Now my calendar was crammed with an assortment of medical and other health-related appointments and my daily naps. I had to take my post-chemo blackout days into account. Everyone knew that any plans I dared make were tentative at best.

I didn't set out to write the Healing Journey letters as "therapy." I simply wrote the first one to let the people in my life know what was happening to me, and to thank those who already knew and who were visiting, calling, and writing. Then the responses started to flood in, with people e-mailing me about how they had appreciated my letter, not just to learn the details of my sobering news but also because I had brought them into the experience of what I was living through. Some wrote to say that my writing had touched them deeply, that it was unusual to be allowed in to what is often a cloistered world in this way, and they were grateful that I had opened the door and let them in. The heartfelt quality of the responses and my desire to put down and share the meanderings of my physical and emotional journey spurred me to want to write more.

I had always longed to put aside time for writing. I had written at work and penned letters, poems, and new lyrics to old tunes all for as long as I can remember. But life had intervened, and, despite my persistent yearnings, I hadn't been in a place where I was willing or able to take the time for a major writing project. Until now.

I was astonished by the urgency I suddenly felt in relation to time during my cancer experience, especially since I wasn't pressured by the demands that had consumed me in the past. Almost every day, I retreated to write in the room on the third floor that I had claimed as my own. Maybe it was my sudden realization about the fleetingness of life, but I felt compelled to "get it all down" right away. For the first time, I allowed my writing to become deeply personal. I wanted to create a chronicle of what was happening to me, about what I was thinking and feeling along the way. As soon as I sent out one of my letters, I'd begin the next one, even if I didn't finish it for another few weeks.

I sometimes lost myself in the writing, unaware of what time it was. I'd forget to eat or to take a nap. When I wasn't writing, I constantly thought about the things I was working on, turning over sentences in my mind, coming up with new ideas, trying out better ways to express them. If there were too many things happening in my day, I resented that I wasn't getting my writing time in. I felt compelled to get back to it.

When I was writing, I was anxious and on edge but grounded at the same time. It was a strange new paradox but an enormously satisfying one. I realized that the writing was becoming "therapy" (Greek for *healing*) in its best sense because it was helping me to both quell my terrors and make sense of the changes happening in my body and in my life. As my writing grew to become my consistent "work," I began to think that it was also becoming an essential part of what might heal me.

I took on a second writing project: a correspondence with my mother. My mom was a seasoned letter writer, and her letters to and from her friend Oonagh Berry had been published in the book *Between Friends: A Year in Letters* several years before. I had admired their discipline and courage to write openly about their lives.

My mom and I had often talked about starting a correspondence, but hadn't managed to make it happen. But when I started chemo, we decided that now was the time. We would write a letter to each other every three weeks. She would write in longhand and I'd write on the computer, then we would send our letters in the mail. There would be no requirement to specifically respond to each other's letters, just to write from our hearts. We decided to call our correspondence project "58/85" – our respective ages at the time.

In one of my first letters, I wrote:

> There's no doubt that this newly found spaciousness I have so long craved has a lot to do with making this writing possible. But did I have to get sick for it to happen??? I remember having a glimpse of it when we were on strike a few years ago. The strike was hard in lots of ways, with minus 30-degree temperatures in February, picket duty several times a week, and no pay. But the amazing thing was that we couldn't, weren't allowed to, do any work. It meant that not only was there free time when I wasn't

picketing, but that my mind and spirit were free to go places they hadn't explored before. I didn't write then, but I distinctly recall the feeling of being open to the possibility in a way that had previously eluded me.

Now, in the midst of this scourge, it has become part of the letting go because it's clear and because I have no choice, like when I was on strike. And now that it's here, I realize how hungry – starved – I was for it, and how voraciously I'm consuming it. But why didn't I give myself permission to make it a choice before now?

My mom and I wrote only two letters to each other that fall before another catastrophe struck our family. But the correspondence was a rich and meaningful experience for both of us. It wouldn't be until the following summer that we would resume again.

The 58/85 correspondence with my now eighty-eight-year-old mom carries on. Although there are times when her hand is shaky and it is physically difficult for her to put pen to paper, we remain deeply committed to writing our letters. Writing means building a quiet space into our lives where we shut out distraction and focus on expressing what we're thinking and doing in our lives at a new level. Among other explorations, we continue to navigate "the country of old age," from our different vantage points. Our letters have become yet another way into our relationship, and we both hungrily look forward to the letters in our mailboxes.

Living with a catastrophic illness and going through treatment require us to slow down, even to stop completely sometimes. This is a major adjustment for most of us, especially if we have been high functioning "doers." We have to figure out who we are if we're not actively engaging with the world. We also have to let go of our former ways as we determine, possibly for the first time, how to "be."

"Being" is a foreign concept for many of us in the western world and certainly for social activists. We associate "just being" with sloth, and feel guilty if we're not doing or accomplishing something. It was something I had worked on with Joyce many years before cancer. I had been doing too much and my sense of self was too dependent on what I was doing. While I mostly enjoyed each of the activities I undertook, there were simply too many of them. I wasn't able to savor each activity because there wasn't enough space between them. Napping, one of my favorite indulgences, eluded me. Joyce talked to me about "spaciousness," about the abundance that can flow our way if we take steps to consciously "aerate" our lives.

Although the idea of spaciousness had lots of appeal, I was a painfully slow learner. When I was diagnosed, Joyce reminded me that now more than ever, I would need to let myself rest and "be." In fact, it would be an essential part of my healing.

When we are ill and going through treatment, we become "patients" who require a great deal of "patience" as we wait, sometimes for seemingly interminable amounts of time. We wait for our test results in our doctors' offices, for our side effects to subside, for the next phase of our treatment to begin, for our treatment to be over. As we wait or as we appear to be idle, we may find that it is in these in-between times where we have the possibility of finding a new sense of spaciousness.

Like winter, the spaces between can give the illusion that nothing is happening. But dormancy is deceptive both in the natural world and within ourselves, and is an essential phase of the life cycle. Like dormancy, spaciousness is deeply generative, a place from which our richest creativity and growth can emerge.

Spaciousness came slowly following my diagnosis. It certainly didn't present itself while I was wandering in the wilderness searching for a treatment plan. But with Joyce's help, it started to emerge and ultimately blossom.

It takes different forms for each of us. It might express itself in art, music, in creations of wood, fabric or yarn, or other creative endeavor. I believe my writing flowed from that generative place. Or it may not result in anything tangible we "produce" other than a new sense of being in the world. Whatever it is, our spaces between can be a time of opportunity for transformation, one that we hope to carry forward into our lives beyond cancer.

CHAPTER FOUR

Coming Undone:
Finding Strength in Vulnerability

I was in the thick of treatment, the thick of misery. An unrelenting, debilitating cough had gripped me, keeping me writhing for hours each night as I tossed and turned under the covers, wracked by convulsions and heaving. I'd have fitful bouts of sleep and get up exhausted and spent. I somehow lumbered around the house semi-upright through the day by consuming gallons of hot water mixed with lemon juice and honey, but I dreaded going to bed. My cough persisted into what normally would have been the "good" two weeks of my three-week chemo cycle, and, frustrated, I had to cancel almost everything that I had planned for this time.

It was discouraging to realize the extent to which my immune system had been weakened by chemo and that my natural resistance was so depleted. I was disappointed not to be able to indulge in simple pleasures: walking with Denise, going to the Y, having short visits with friends or with my parents. Talking on the phone was almost impossible. I had little interest in eating much of anything. With my head in a fog, it was hard to focus on reading the newspaper or a book. It was all I could do to drag myself to my desk to write for short snatches of time.

I had been looking forward to an Arlo Guthrie concert at a downtown church. When the time came I didn't know if I could go because of my cough, but it was a rare outing and we had already bought our tickets. Larry and I headed out, armed with a thermos of hot toddy and pockets full of cough drops and tissues. The concert was fabulous, with Arlo, his kids, and grandchildren belting out many of my favorite songs, but I hated not to be able to sing or even croak along. I was a wretched basket case throughout the show, and I felt badly for the people sitting near me as I hacked and sputtered through the evening. I must have been quite a sight, ashen-faced and bleary-eyed in my black bandana, doubled over in fits of coughing on the hard wooden pew.

My cough presented other problems. I'd finally had my cumbersome PICC line removed after my last chemo session and had an appointment to have a portocath inserted. It would involve minor surgery by a radiologist who would insert the device into my chest, attaching it to my vein so that I could receive chemo safely. But how could they possibly insert the portocath into my chest if I was still coughing up a storm? If I didn't have the portocath, I couldn't go to my next round of chemo because the chemicals were too toxic to inject directly into my vein.

A virulent strain of the flu bug, H1N1, was circulating, felling otherwise healthy people and even causing some deaths. Vaccination sites were being set up across the province. In the early days, there was a question of whether cancer patients should receive the vaccine because of our already weakened immune systems. Eventually, the oncology team at the Cancer Centre agreed that we should be immunized toward the end of our chemo cycles when we were likely to have better resistance. Although I had never had a flu shot before, I decided to get it this time because of cancer. But did it make sense for me to have it with my cough?

So far, I hadn't needed to miss a chemo session because my white blood cell counts had been all right. Now I was worried I might not make it to my next round. A delay in chemo would have a domino effect, delaying the remainder of my rounds. The year-long duration of my treatment already felt interminable. In the end, thanks to some heavy-duty narcotic cough syrup prescribed by my family doctor, the cough abated after three awful weeks. It seemed like a miracle that I was able to get the vaccine, my portocath was inserted as planned, and I went through my fourth round of chemo on schedule. I was relieved to be halfway through the chemo. But the experience brought home how fragile and vulnerable I was. I couldn't make any assumptions about where the cancer or my treatment would take me. I couldn't make assumptions about anything in my life.

✉ Healing Journey #4

___

November 12, 2009

Dear friends and family,

This has been a discouraging time. Last week we got the devastating news that my father, Gil, is gravely ill. Other than a bout with prostate cancer eight years ago and abdominal surgery in 2008, my dad has always been strong and healthy: he has a strong constitution, he didn't smoke or drink, and was a regular at the gym, on the tennis court, etc. After several days of feeling terribly weak, he has now been admitted to hospital with acute leukemia. It makes me crazy that I can't even visit him there because of the danger of my catching the H1N1 flu virus.

Things don't look good for him. It feels like it's too much for one family to bear.

It's hard not to think about longevity, old age, and mortality in new ways these days. I used to imagine that I'd probably live a long life because I was strong and healthy, exercised, and ate well and because there seemed to be longevity genes in my family. I'd talk with friends about how we would try to "do" old age differently than our parents' generation, that we would create "feminaries" and six-plexes where we would live independently and communally and support each other as we aged.

At the Blue Skies Music festival a couple of years ago, some of us went to a workshop on "Aging Courageously." We came away with lots of ideas on how to age both consciously and well. At this summer's Blue Skies, I mused about proposing a workshop for next year's program on "Writing Your Own Epitaph," which would of course be much more to do with making choices about how we live than dying and tombstones.

On the subject of mortality, I had a sobering moment a couple of weeks ago when I went to a meditation class at Breast Cancer Action, a local survivor-led group that supports breast cancer patients and their families. I'd been looking forward to it, to being with other women who are going through or have been through breast cancer. Besides, it was a way to learn about meditation at the same time. I'm not sure what I was expecting, but I was surprised when I arrived to see that all the other women there had hair! While some were in remission, several were living with metastatic cancer that had spread from their original breast cancer. That was the scary part. One woman who had been diagnosed with breast cancer nineteen years ago at the age of twenty-eight had undergone treatment and was cancer-free until it returned when she was forty-four. She is going through chemo again now and is fighting nausea, etc., but as the cancer is in her bones this time, the chemo is not the kind that makes her lose her hair. It was a whole new aspect of "survival" I hadn't thought about much until now. Survival doesn't necessarily mean being cancer-free. It just means being alive.

I'm still wrestling with the chemo paradox: How do I reconcile the awful side effects of chemotherapy with the positive benefits of its healing? At a dream class that I signed up for at a local yoga center, a dream I had had inspired me to create this dialogue between my "strong" self and the self that is feeling sick and weak.

Weak self: I need your care and compassion to get through this difficult time.

Strong self: I find it hard to do that, because you're so unfamiliar to me. I'm not usually tolerant of weakness, especially in myself.

Weak self: You may not be able to see it yet, but I can open new doors for you.

Strong self: What doors?

Weak self: The door to vulnerability, of allowing yourself

to be cared for, of finding time and space for reflection, for deepening your intuition. These are things I know you have long yearned for, some of the gifts I can give you.

Strong self: How?

Weak self: You have to slow down and notice me, see what I can offer. You must cherish and nurture me not out of pity, but as a part of yourself that you value, treasure, and love and who will be part of finding your true and authentic self.

Strong self: Is there anything else?

Weak self: I am the path to healing and to being well again. I am also the path to the next chapter of your life, one that will take you into healthy, vibrant aging. You ignore me at your peril. Will you walk with me?

Figuring out that both my strong and weak selves are essential to my healing has helped me accept my vulnerability as an important part of getting well.

While this has been a discouraging time, there have still been precious moments:

- Walking in the crunching leaves on the sunny blackout days (talk about paradox!) of last weekend with Karen and Rachel when I felt okay enough

- Receiving your e-mails saying that what I have written about has resonated with something in your life

- Opening a package to discover a gorgeous hand-knitted vest of many colors and three funky wool hats from Edna in Calgary

- In spite of my cough, being at an Inter Pares board meeting with support, back-up, and love from staff and fellow board members

- Cindy coming to chemo with me when Larry was sick
- Being part of a new book club of terrific women hell-bent on creativity and irreverence
- Debbie and Denise organizing the "Supper Sisters," the wonderful team of women who bring us yummy meals on chemo Thursdays and Saturdays
- Singing with the Havurah band on a glorious Sunday afternoon
- Ellen and Anne-Marie planning a healing circle for me
- Having my first shower after a workout at the Y (instead of at home) with my new portocath
- Receiving a fat, handwritten, heartfelt letter from my mom via snail mail as part of our 58/85 letter writing project
- Hearing that Missy Burgess dedicated her show at the Black Sheep to raise money for the healing garden for cancer patients (I couldn't be there because of my cough)
- Daniel organizing my array of naturopathic supplements into a color-coded pill box every week
- Larry playing Upwords with me and giving me head rubs

Nathan told me about his friend whose goal at the end of breast cancer treatment was to swim with the dolphins, and about how important it was for her to keep her "eye on the prize." For a woman in my support group who had breast cancer for the second time, it was to see Elton John in Las Vegas.

I was thinking about what my "prize" could be when a beautiful card and a pair of earrings from Sue arrived all the way from the Greek island of Santorini. I'd always wanted to go the Greek islands. The brilliant blue water and white buildings of Sue's card, and later her spectacular photographs and stories of her time there cemented the dream: my goal is to go to the Greek Islands when my active treatment is over.

Once again, thank you from the bottom of my heart for your letters, e-mail messages, calls, cards, and gifts from near and far. I want you to know that your love and support mean the world to me.

Be well. Carpe diem.
Love, Tamara

Reflections

ANOTHER FAMILY HEARTBREAK

On my birthday a few months before I was diagnosed, my dad, the quintessential researcher, asked me, "How many fifty-eight-year-olds do you know who have two parents in relatively good shape?" Sadly, I could hardly think of anyone else.

In my family, my father had always been our Gibraltar, the guy you could count on to be there. He still had a strong constitution, and with a few blips, had been hale and hearty throughout most of his life. He'd played tennis, cycled, and gone to the gym regularly until a year before. He loved life and there was so much he still wanted to do. He often said he planned to live to be 120 years old, as in the old Jewish blessing that you should live as long and as well as Moses.

At the end of October, my dad was at the cottage with Larry and Daniel cutting up dead trees, reveling in the glory of his "prima" season of brilliant fall colors – especially the reds, his favorite. A week later he suddenly became terribly weak, saw his doctor, and had blood tests done. The diagnosis was acute leukemia and my father was admitted to hospital. We were in shock.

I was devastated that on top of everything else, I couldn't visit him because I was considered vulnerable to disease. When we first talked on the phone, he vowed that, "we'd walk shoulder to shoulder" through our treatments together.

It was a huge relief to finally get permission from Dr. Verma to visit my dad. When I found his room, he was alone in bed, his stubbled face ashen and gray. I approached and leaned over, reaching to hold his head and kiss his damp forehead, squeezing his fingers tightly as I looked long into his eyes. With his brow furrowed and his voice quavering, his mind was still working hard. He struggled to tell me how it had all happened so fast. "It's over," he conceded. "There isn't anything they can do for me."

He could no longer get out of bed to sit in a wheelchair or get to the bathroom. My resilient and optimistic father had become weak and debilitated. I was relieved when he said that he wasn't in pain; the doctors were taking care of that. I told him I loved him, how he'd been a great dad, and how I'd hated not being able to visit him.

As I fed him ice chips for his parched lips, my father listed the names of the people he wanted to see: the three grandchildren, a few close friends, two special cousins. A long-time lover of folk music, he listened to friend and troubadour Chris sing and play some of his favorites. He even talked about the songs he wanted at his memorial. My dad told me he was disappointed he wouldn't be able to go through cancer treatment alongside me. He said he hoped I'd beat my cancer.

I had spoken to Dr. Verma about my father's leukemia and found out that for my dad, treatment would have been far worse than the cancer. We all knew there would have been nothing worse than to see him go through treatment that would have tortured him before it killed him. My dad agreed to have a DO NOT RESUSCITATE sign put at the head of his bed.

My dad was dying, and I was faced with yet another reminder of my own mortality. I was anguished to watch him while I was in the grips of my own cancer. It was the first time I'd been so near a person I loved as he was dying, watching the dwindling and then the expiring of such a powerful life force. It was as if I was witnessing it with my hands tied behind my back, looking on as a once-raging fire was reduced to smoldering logs and then cold embers. I thought: *This is what death looks like, a preview. Are you ready?*

In a strange way, death became more knowable in the process. I was becoming familiar with its pallor and smell, its cunning and idiosyncrasies. Its presence in my life had become more commonplace and thus less terrifying, even less imminent. I imagined that if I were to befriend death as a regular player in my life, I might be able to defang it, even bring it to its knees for a while. As every cancer patient knows, death will always stalk us. But if I could keep it at bay for now, outside my perimeter for whatever in-between time I had, it might give me some added force for living my life.

> **Joyce Hardman:** There is a point where you have to accept that the mystery might include the death of your body and make peace with it. When you make peace with the mystery and then you keep walking more bravely into it, the idea of your mortality is no longer terrifying. It loosens up a freedom to live.

SLOWING DOWN: AGING AND LONGEVITY

Before cancer, I hadn't spent a lot of time thinking about aging and longevity. Like my dad, I'd presumed longevity because it ran in my family. Over the years, Larry and I had developed some common assumptions about how our lives and deaths would unfold. Larry was eight years older than I, he was a longtime smoker, and he didn't have much longevity in his family. We both imagined he'd die first and that I'd be widowed. He'd long been encouraging me to join him in retirement. He said he wanted us to have time together and explore the world while we were still healthy. I looked forward to those things too, but I knew I wasn't ready to stop working yet.

I wasn't afraid of aging. I had positive examples around me of my parents and a grandmother who had aged well. While I imagined being older as a time of slowing down, I also saw myself singing, swimming, and living in some kind of supportive community decades down the road. I didn't think a lot about infirmity and loneliness.

But cancer changed everything. I could no longer presume anything about the future: going back to work, anticipating the adventures of retirement, maybe becoming a grandmother someday, organizing creative living situations, getting old with its attendant joys and hardships. Instead, the real possibility that I could be approaching the end of my life had come so close I could taste it. The uncharted trajectory of my cancer could mean that I'd be "untimely ripp'd" from my life and from the world before I turned sixty. My father's looming death was another reminder of my vulnerability, the fragility of life, and the unknown future.

I think I was pretty smug about presuming my longevity. While it's useful to imagine ways to live well long into the future, I wonder now about what longevity really means. Surely it's not just about living to be 100 – we all know people who are miserable in their old age and want their lives to end. Perhaps longevity is more about finding ways to slow down, to make each day count; about choosing with our hearts; and savoring each experience, encounter, and relationship we have. The irony was that, just as I was coming to grips with the prospect of dying, I was also starting to discover some new clues to the secret of longevity. It was poignantly clear that this period of my life was going to be a time out on many levels. It would be my winter.

Joyce asked me at one point about my relationship with the seasons. She asked me, if spring is about planting (initiating), if summer is about growing (nurturing and tending), if fall is about harvesting (focusing on the product) and winter is about fallow time and regeneration (valuing reflection), which did I "do" well? Which did I need to work on?

I knew the answer right away: I was pretty good at all the seasons – except winter. While I loved winter and knew the value of dormancy and regeneration, literally and metaphorically, I realized that in my life and work I was often guilty of ignoring or diminishing its rightful place in the natural cycle. Once the harvest was done, I'd usually start new projects before I took the time to breathe, reflect, and recoup.

Now, I had no choice. Sometimes I stopped completely. I wasn't living in the past or the future, only in the present. The dark times I spent recovering from chemo and the countless hours I spent in hospital waiting rooms, the in-between times and spaces, allowed me to notice what was around and within me in new ways. With my mind on high alert, I was constantly processing all that was happening to me.

During treatment, I was never bored. I was keenly aware of my body, how it felt, how it looked, how well or badly it was functioning, when it was "on" or "off." My senses were heightened. I saw the sky, heard the birds, and listened to music differently, finding myself more sharply attuned to nuance, texture, and tone. As the spaces between my activities grew wider, it seemed that new openings and possibilities were starting to emerge.

I asked myself: why did I let my work, etc., consume me to the point that I couldn't/didn't let spaciousness happen? Why hadn't I practiced my mom's "vacuum" strategy of consciously deciding not to fill in the gaps and spaces in the hope that others would fill them in? I was lousy enough about creating emotional and practical vacuums so others would fill them, but I wasn't even able to create vacuums for myself in my work or personal life. In the midst of cancer, it became part of the letting go because I had no choice. Now that I had to slow down, I realized how hungry I had been for it, and how voraciously I was consuming it. Why hadn't I given myself permission to make it a choice before? Did I need to get sick to figure it out? Was this one of the "gifts" of going through cancer?

I promised myself that if I were to get well, I would live my life in new ways. I would live slower and with more spaciousness, and thus live "longer" in the best sense. I would reclaim my winter.

DREAM WORK

One of the new things I'd decided to do during treatment was to sign up for a dream class. It was a major departure for me. I wasn't into yoga, and I wasn't especially good at remembering my dreams. I wondered whether I'd find it hokey. One of the attractions of the class was that it involved keeping a journal, which I thought might be a good way to inspire my writing. Two friends who had had breast cancer had found the class a useful way to explore deeply what was going on for them. I decided to try it.

When I arrived for the first class, a few people were already gathered in a circle. They welcomed me before beginning to chant to the droning sounds of the harmonium played by the lone man, the scent of incense wafting through the air. I was clearly the newcomer; everyone else seemed familiar with the drill. After the chanting, one of the leaders invited me to step aside with her to find out how the class worked.

She explained that the others had been meeting for years. Our task was to remember our dreams, and write down what we recalled in our journals as soon as we woke up, even if it was the middle of the night. The chanting help us move into a meditative state, where we would be more likely to access the meaning of our dreams. We were to bring our dream journals to class, where the leaders would use various techniques to help us understand and make use of what our dreams were telling us about our lives. If we chose to, we could share our insights.

I came back and joined the group. When they invited me to introduce myself, I took a deep breath and said I was going through treatment for breast cancer and hoped the dream class would bring me new insights. The group responded warmly, and I decided to put my scepticism aside to explore what dream work was about. If it was going to help me explore the recesses of my sub-conscious self, I would have to be open to the chanting and to a language that invoked "light" and "mother."

The amazing thing was that as the weeks went on, I started to remember parts of my dreams as never before. I wrote down what I could recall, and brought the dream fragments to class. With the help of the leaders and the more seasoned "dreamers," I learned new ways to look at my dreams and how to connect them with what was going on in the rest of my life.

The dream I wrote about in my fourth letter spoke to one of the paradoxes I was starting to uncover as I traveled through my journey with cancer. In the dream, Larry and I are driving in the countryside through fields and meadows with no particular destination. We come upon some of the people who work in the basement of my workplace, in shipping and receiving, the print shop, etc. They are some of the most human, down-to-earth, and likeable people at work. They ask me how I'm doing and when I'm coming back to work. I miss them and I'm feeling pretty good at the moment, so I say that I think I'll probably be coming back to work soon. Then I look back at Larry, who is grimacing and motioning for me to say no, that I won't be coming back. I realize that I'm in one of my two good post-chemo weeks, that there are lots of other times when I feel wretched and sick, and that more terrors await me around the corner. I tell them I'm sorry, that I've made a terrible mistake, and that I won't be coming back for a long time.

When I brought this dream to class, one of the tasks was to identify the many "I"s in the dream, and to figure out whether the particular "I" was active or passive. Then we wrote a dialogue between the two separate "I"s and came up with what they would say to each other. My dialogue was between the strong "I" and the "I" that is sick, weak, and vulnerable. My weaker self tries to convince my stronger self that it has something worthwhile to offer, that it needs love and attention, that it is the key to intimacy. It too has gifts. Perhaps it holds the key to my healing.

I didn't know much about how the subconscious mind reveals itself through dreams, but during the months I attended the dream class, I was intrigued by the glimpses of how it worked. Certainly, the dream about my stronger and weaker selves provided an insight into how, if I embraced my vulnerability, it could play an important role in my healing. In the midst of upheaval, understanding my dreams was another way to pay attention to what was going on.

> **Joyce Hardman:** It's an amazing experience that happens ten times larger with a critical illness because the whole experience is condensed. The people who are being treated for cancer and are healing have left their daily lives, their habits, their jobs, their routines behind. As a result, they've come undone and that undoneness is powerful. With other clients, I'm always trying to joggle them into a bit more undoneness so they can see a larger vista. But it's a lot harder for them than with someone who is dealing with cancer.

HEALING THROUGH VULNERABILITY

Like most who grow up in our culture, I was encouraged to be strong and capable, to excel and succeed in my personal and public worlds. To some extent, it appeared that I had "succeeded." But I also knew at some level that the push to be strong and successful was a cruel hoax, an illusion that badly covered up our inevitable frailties. In the process, it denied our humanness, keeping us apart from each other instead of bringing us together. I wondered: if we could be honest about our weaknesses and our vulnerabilities, would we be more likely to be closer and more supportive of one another? If we asked questions rather than thinking we had to have the answers, could we find more authentic connections? If we could find ways to relate to each other more honestly, wouldn't we be stronger for it?

I had spent the last twenty plus years doing literacy and popular education work in the labor movement. Unions champion workers' rights, stand up for the underdog, and work for social change. But for the most part, they carry on within a macho culture where they are in constant fighting mode. Showing weaknesses or not knowing the answers are generally seen as signs of failure. There are exceptions, the fertile pockets where brave souls seek out "spaces of freedom" and try different ways of working, learning, and relating. But generally, it is a work environment where taking risks and showing vulnerability isn't easy. Now I lacked the trappings of "strength" in the usual sense. I was no longer working at my job, so I had no status or "outside" identity in the world. I had been stripped, reduced to being my raw, unvarnished self.

Joyce Hardman: Helplessness is feeling like "I don't know how the heck this happened to me, I was trying to do everything right." It means going through all kinds of treatments that make no sense to the heart or the body yet that's what is out there for us. You have no idea of what the outcome will be and little or no control over who your healers are. You're walking through helplessness all over the place.

My dream about strength and weakness was instructive. In this state of life-threatening vulnerability, I was astonished to uncover a new kind of strength. If I felt safe with someone, I could talk openly about what was happening to me, without needing to hide or protect my fallibilities. I could talk about cancer, the trauma of losing my hair, the lethargy and queasiness of my blackout days, my fears. If I extended an invitation into my world, those who chose to enter it could come through a door that was wide open.

Sometimes, those I shared my stories with said they were grateful to have the chance to be brought into my experience. Often, they were vaguely familiar with cancer but didn't know it intimately, as it had so often been hidden from view. They told me my letters helped them understand what the experience was about in new ways. They said they had gained new empathy for the people close to them whose lives had been stricken by cancer but who were unwilling or unable to share what they were living through. It also dawned on me that in exposing my own underbelly, people were in turn able to respond with stories of their own infirmities, fears, and vulnerabilities; their moments of bumbling and awkwardness. Often, the bond between us would deepen to a new level.

It wasn't just about cancer. While there is no doubt cancer was a dominant theme, I was determined not to let it become the sum total of me. When friends called or visited, I didn't want the conversation to be just about me or cancer. Sometimes, they felt that what was going on in their lives was trivial in comparison. But I always asked how they were doing, wanting to hear about their lives too, insisting we talk about other things. Usually, I sensed they were relieved, glad to offer up their stories of family, work, their adventures and misadventures.

LEARNING TO RECEIVE

When we feel we need to be strong or at least appear to be so, it can be difficult to accept offers of support or practical help with open arms. After all, if we're powerful and self-reliant, who needs help? Sometimes, the newly diagnosed patient isn't ready or able to receive, and she'll resist or refuse offers of support. There may be people in her life who she doesn't feel comfortable having around her, especially in her altered, unpredictable, and vulnerable state. She may be wary of intrusion as she draws a tight circle around the few she is willing to let into her increasingly private and reclusive world, one where she feels safer and more secure. She may not yet understand that choosing to receive can be a gift, and that her vulnerability and even her helplessness can bring her abundant love and strength. She can learn that by allowing herself to receive and thus be loved, she will gain true strength.

Joyce Hardman: For most of the women I see, being in a receiving role is not their usual domain. They have jobs and other roles where they're much more in control.

During my early days of treatment, my friends Debbie and Denise announced they were coming over, arriving on my doorstep armed with notebooks, calendars, and ideas, ready to roll up their sleeves. As the three of us sat around my dining room table drinking green tea, they put it on the table. They wanted to know what I needed help with, what they could do for me, and when. They offered to cook, organize my home office, make phone calls, do Internet research, and drive me to appointments. They offered to recruit and co-ordinate support from other people.

Their generosity touched me deeply. But I didn't know what would be helpful from one day to the next, so I was at a loss to know how to respond. I found it difficult to plan: I had recently started chemo and didn't know what lay ahead, how I would feel or what I would want or need in the coming weeks. I was too overwhelmed to think about what it would mean to fit in outside "help" on top of everything else.

Food was complicated: I had little interest in eating in the days following chemo. I was, however, able to enjoy eating during the two weeks that followed. But would I be imposing on my friends? Whose names would I suggest? Would they feel required to participate? What if they didn't like to cook? I found it difficult to ask for help, but I knew I had to get over my reluctance and find a way to accept the support on offer.

Debbie and Denise forged ahead and came up with a plan. What about having suppers prepared and delivered every Sunday and on chemo Thursdays? Did I have any food issues? How many would be eating? (I said healthy food with no red meat or deep-fried food, no desserts, and enough for Larry, Daniel, and me would be great.) Later, in the spring when I went through radiation, they started the meals again and added rides to the hospital. Friends who didn't enjoy cooking could choose to drive. All I had to do was to come up with a list of names and e-mail addresses. They took care of the rest.

It wasn't hard to put the list together, but I still doubted whether they really meant it, if it would come together, and if I deserved so much love. Debbie and Denise composed an e-mail message to send

Joyce Hardman: We can't know how our life will unfold, but we can set out general intentions and wishes. As we accept our helplessness, we often find that the world rises up, because it does again and again in ways that surprise you, that love you beyond how you can love yourself.

out asking for volunteers to sign on as a "Supper Sister" to bring meals on specific dates over the next five months. Within a day or two, my doubts ebbed.

I wasn't in on the e-mail exchange, but Debbie and Denise told me there was a flurry of messages back and forth within the group. Many had written to say they were grateful to have a way to help out and give me practical support. In no time, the supper slots were taken, with some friends even complaining that they hadn't got their name into a slot in time!

As the suppers started to arrive, I realized that what was being created was about much more than the food. Each meal was lovingly and thoughtfully prepared, presented, and delivered. Some even arrived with menus, flowers, and candles! If I was up for it, I'd have a short visit with the cook, an added bonus. When Larry, Daniel, and I sat down to eat, we savored every spoonful of delicious soup, each morsel of roasted chicken or pasta or organic vegetables. It helped me feel nurtured and cared for, truly well "fed."

CHAPTER FIVE

Mortality:
Grieving and Moving Forward

In what felt like a heartbeat, my dad succumbed to the ravages of acute leukemia. I badly needed to grieve for him, to find quiet time to try to make sense of what had happened and come to terms with living in a world without my dad. I also had to find a way to soldier on in my fight, and allow myself to imagine life after losing my dad. I just had to get through this crazy time.

I had known the local folk singer Missy Burgess for a few years, but we became closer while planning my dad's memorial where she sang and played with other musicians who had known him. I loved her music, both the old songs she sang and the new ones she composed. Missy had lost two close friends to cancer, and had performed at benefits to raise money to create healing gardens in hospitals for cancer patients. I was thrilled when she offered to come to the cancer center to sing me through my next chemo session.

Here was yet another paradox: how could we sing through chemo, especially with the dreaded toxic chemicals running through my veins? I'd seen other patients in the chemo room listening to music through their headphones, but it had always been a solitary thing. This would be out in the open, a public happening. Missy's offer was a crazy, fantastic idea. I needed to go through chemo anyway, so why not make it as positive an experience as possible? Maybe the other patients and their families would enjoy it too. But would the hospital allow it?

A new chemo area had just opened. It was in a different configuration from the old fish bowl. Now several pods were laid out in a circle like the petals of a flower. There were six beds and a nursing station in each pod, with natural light pouring in the windows. There was lots of room and plenty of visitors' chairs around the beds. The new space seemed calmer, more spacious, and less chaotic. Maybe it would even be a place for singing.

When I saw Dr. Verma a couple of days before chemo, I asked the receptionist if Missy could come to sing during my upcoming session. She called over the head nurse, who thought it would be all right as long as the music was acoustic and not too loud, and the other patients weren't bothered by it. On a snowy December morning, Larry and I picked up Missy and her guitar and headed for the hospital.

As the nurse set me up on the bed, Missy made the rounds of the other patients in my pod. A former nurse with a big, outgoing personality and a hearty laugh, she introduced herself to the patients, their families, and the nurses, learning their names and finding out what kind of music they liked. Then she pulled out her guitar and started to sing.

It's hard to describe what it was like to receive chemo and sing at the same time. It felt right: strong, defiant, and life affirming. As we sang, I closed my eyes and imagined that the poison in the chemo was transforming into a river of light running through my veins. It was healing me: the red angel was trumping the red devil this time. Belting out the harmonies felt joyous, triumphant, even fun. Other patients called out their requests and joined in the singing. The time was over before we knew it. I was delighted when Missy offered to come again for my last two rounds of chemo.

✉ Healing Journey #5

January 27, 2010

Dear friends and family,
The past couple of months have felt like an eternity in so many ways. In the last letter, I wrote about how devastated we were that my father had been diagnosed with acute leukemia. The cancer rampaged through his body like an avalanche, so that even his doctors were surprised at how fast it advanced. Thankfully, though his body failed rapidly and his speech was increasingly belabored, his mind was sharp until the end. He died on the morning of November 16th. Our world changed irrevocably that day.

One could say that my dad had a "good death." He had lived a long and productive life in mostly excellent health. He had loved his work in the union. He had loved his family. He hadn't suffered long, and had his faculties until the end. He had few regrets if any. He'd had superb care in the hospital. He had been able to say goodbye to the people who mattered most to him. The outpouring of love, respect, and gratitude in the letters, cards, e-mails, and phone calls that arrived following word of his illness and then his death, including warm messages from so many of you, was nothing short of phenomenal.

It's all true, but it doesn't tell the whole story. It doesn't tell how much my dad loved life and how he would have given anything for a few more years to live it well. (Four days before he died, after he was already in palliative care at the hospital, he asked his doctor if there was anywhere in the world he could go for treatment. If there had been a chance for hope somewhere, I know he would have gone.) It doesn't tell us about the gaping hole left behind that's like an amputated limb, constantly reminding us of his presence and of the pain of losing him long after he's gone. No matter how old we are, we are still orphaned when we lose the father or mother who has always been there for us. Time may heal the sharpness of the pain, but there is no one who can replace my father, ever.

A secular Jew, my dad didn't want a funeral. He had chosen to be cremated and to have his ashes spread around the now towering maple my mom had planted for his seventieth birthday. Two days after he died, on an unusually warm, sunny and windless November day, we spread his ashes in a circle around the tree as he had wished. We gathered afterward to remember him and to read a couple of poems and a story he loved from A *Treasury of Jewish Folklore*.

My mom decided not to sit shiva, the Jewish ritual where friends and family gather at the home of the bereaved after a death to grieve and remember. She wanted to grieve more privately and to focus on the upcoming memorial instead. But I found myself yearning for some kind of collective mourning that would happen sooner rather than later, and talked about it with Judy and Debbie. Within a few days, a group of my women friends and my mom were gathered at Judy's house to remember my dad, to share stories, and of course to sing. It was like a big group hug and an important step in my grieving process.

We chose December 12th for Dad's memorial to fit into my chemo schedule and because we wanted it to happen before the holidays. If we hadn't figured it out already, it became abundantly clear that going the non-traditional route outside the usual prescriptions of synagogues, funeral homes, etc., meant that planning the event would be far more emotional and labor-intensive than the usual fare. My dad had also been a master of organizing "program," so we knew he would be watching with a supportive but critical eye as we put the memorial together.

The Canadian Union of Public Employees (CUPE) generously offered to hold the memorial in the atrium of its new national building and to help with graphic design, printing, food, logistics, etc. It was a fitting venue, as my dad had been the research director of

CUPE and its predecessor for thirty-one years, and was still very much part of the union long into his retirement. The only problem was that the atrium could hold a maximum of two hundred people.

We worked hard to have hosts and speakers at the memorial who represented the different parts of my dad's life: his work, his family, his friendships, his passions. Moving tributes were interspersed with the songs he loved, performed by several musician friends with the rest of us singing along. My cousin Sara sang a beautiful Yiddish song *a cappella*. Rachel did us proud with her heartfelt tribute to her grandfather that brought both laughter and tears. I didn't know whether Karen and I would get through our tribute and poem without breaking down, but in the end, the memorial was more than we ever could have hoped for. My dad, the quintessential organizer, had brought people together yet again, and we all loved him for it.

We were exhausted after the memorial, as it had been a flat-out job planning it for almost a month. It was wonderful, but it had consumed our energies to the point that we weren't able to take the time to do the slow, quiet grieving we desperately needed to do. After consulting the kids, we canceled Chanukah and just spent family time together over the holidays. I found myself looking forward to January, when the holidays would be done with, when I could finally have the time and space to sit inside my grief.

Before my dad died, I had finished the fourth of my eight rounds of chemo. The side effects had been crummy: I was queasy and listless, everything tasted awful, etc. But I had learned what to expect, how to listen to my body, and, for the most part, how to cope and get through it.

The next four rounds were to involve a different drug. I had heard horror stories about docetaxel (Taxotere) from some of the women in my breast cancer support group. It can cause white blood counts to fall steeply, putting us at a high risk of infection. We are instructed to take our temperatures daily. If we develop even a low fever, we are told to go to emergency immediately, where we are given injections to boost our cell counts. A couple of women in my support group ended up in hospital for several days when they were on the drug. One described her pain as being "worse than childbirth," like she was "giving birth to a horse." They also talked about debilitating stomach and bone pain and side effects that included mouth sores, cracked finger and toenails, excessive tearing and crusting of their eyes, and neuropathy that made it difficult to walk.

With these stories racing through my head, I expressed my fears to Dr. Verma. He listened attentively as always, then asked whether I had a drug plan. He said that enough of his patients were ending up in hospital that he had recently started prescribing the drug peg-filgrastim (Neulasta) preventively. Injected by a home care nurse the day after chemo, it would prevent my cell count from dropping and reduce some of the worst side effects. The shots cost $2,800 each, and I would need one for each of the next four rounds of chemo! Thankfully, our drug plans covered the cost, but it is an outrage that there are so many women without drug plans, on Employment Insurance, etc. who do not have the means to buy the drugs they need.

I was still full of trepidation when I went for chemo on November 28th. On a bed for the first time – I had been in a recliner chair for the four rounds – the nurse ominously put ice mitts on my hands and bags of ice on my feet. She explained that they were there to protect my finger and toenails by trying to keep the chemo from reaching my extremities. As the drug dripped into my veins, the nurse checked my vital signs frequently, watching for signs of anaphylactic shock which apparently happens to 2 percent of patients. I tried valiantly to apply my "red angel" healing mantra to the toxins coursing through me, but my struggle with the chemo paradox was harder this time. The chemo was over after a couple of hours, and I went home to wait in dread.

I was mostly okay until Day 6. Then the bone pain set in. When it arrived, it felt like a bulldozer crushing my lower back, pelvis, and legs. I went to bed, for the first time taking the painkiller I had been prescribed, hoping I would sleep until it was over. I got up a couple of hours later, still feeling wretched. My mom came over and stroked my bald head on her lap for hours on the couch. The next day, the pain had mostly receded but my bones felt spongy, as if they weren't solid, and my energy was completely depleted. Even worse, my vision was so blurred that I couldn't read or see well enough to drive safely. The blurred vision was almost more upsetting for me than the pain, a final indignity. The worst of the side effects lasted for about three more days before they finally tapered off.

I was overjoyed at the beginning of November when I finally had a portocath inserted under the skin on my chest for receiving chemo, replacing my wretched PICC line. It meant that I could work out at the Y and then shower unencumbered. The best part, though, was that I would be able to swim, and I started doing laps with a bathing cap absurdly pulled over my bald head for camouflage instead of the uncapped ponytail I used to wear. Sometimes, I'm depleted and can only do a modified workout. It's keeping me in shape, relatively speaking, but I think the Y is also keeping me sane. It continues to evolve from a place of trepidation to one of sanctuary.

One morning, a young woman with shoulder-length hair was in the change room with her guide dog getting ready to go into the pool. She asked whether anyone had an elastic for her ponytail. When I offered her one, she asked whether I needed it for myself. I explained that I didn't have hair because I was going through chemo for breast cancer. She talked about how hard it was for her as a blind person to swim laps with other people in her lane, but was thankful when a couple of women in the pool had asked the lifeguard if she could have her own lane, which made all the difference. An encounter that started out with vulnerability on both sides led to a momentary but powerful connection.

A few days after my father's memorial, it was time for my second round of Taxotere. I was fearful about the side effects after the tough going with the first round, and raised it with Dr. Verma. He suggested taking dexamethasone (Decadron), a powerful steroid, as an antidote for two additional days at half dosage. Although I hated the thought of adding more pharmaceuticals to my body that already felt like a cauldron of chemical soup, I knew his suggestion probably made sense.

Missy Burgess had offered to come with Larry and me to sing and play her guitar through my next round of chemo. I was delighted, and arranged permission with the nurses ahead of time for her to be there. I sang along with Missy as she sat on a stool at the foot of my bed, singing and playing so many of my favorite songs as the drug coursed through my veins. Of course, the other patients, their families, and the nurses loved it too, and I was thrilled when Missy offered to sing me through my remaining rounds of chemo.

My friend Fern had planned to come in from Toronto to help nurse me through the most wretched days. But for the most part, Dr. Verma's idea of taking the extra Decadron worked. I felt crummy but not horrible, depleted, and "off" for a few days. I had spongy bones, fuzzy vision, and excessive tearing but I was able to read and drive. I can't say for sure, but I'm convinced that the complementary therapies I've been doing alongside my medical treatments, which now include intravenous vitamin C, are having an impact. They're helping to fight my cancer but are also lessening the worst side effects of chemo. Even on Taxotere, Fern and I were able to have a pretty good visit, going to a movie, walking, getting to the Y, visiting my mom, and cooking together.

I was moved when two friends offered to plan a healing circle for me. It happened on the winter solstice with a small gathering of women. I felt loved and cared for as we welcomed back the light together. As the year's shortest day dimmed to darkness, we thought about what tomorrow's new light could bring us. After we planted new seeds in pots of moist dark earth, we shared our yearnings for being healthy and told stories over pomegranates and grapes.

In October, I had blood tests to see whether I had the gene mutation that would mean a much higher likelihood of breast cancer recurring. If I tested positive for the gene, I probably would have been advised to have a double mastectomy and have my ovaries removed preventively, and there would have been a 50 percent chance of passing it on to my kids. In December, we got the good news that I don't have the mutated gene. What a huge relief it was for all of us!

For the most part, January has been the quieter month I hoped it would be. The cumulative effect of the chemo has set in, and my endurance and stamina are diminished because of it. As Louise said when she was going through cancer treatment, "*je gueris a plein temps,*" my full-time job is to get well. I still have to go to dozens of medical appointments, and there are tons of things to deal with following my dad's death – I had no idea!

But mostly, I've been trying to be conscious of creating the time and space I need to heal and to grieve. I'm relieved that I've finally started writing again. It fits well with what a friend wrote to me about the next moon cycle called the Bear Moon, which begins on February 13th. On Turtle Island, it is the time when Mama bear gives birth to her cubs deep in her den, emerging a couple of months later. Winter is the season of the Bear, a time to go inward into the darkness.

When I saw Dr. Verma yesterday, he was pleased with my progress. The chemo is working, and the tumors have shrunk by more than 50 percent. After my last round of chemo tomorrow, I'll have an MRI to find out definitively how much the tumors have shrunk and to make sure the cancer hasn't spread. Then there will be a break until my surgery, now scheduled for March 9th, which will involve a lumpectomy and the removal of my lymph nodes. Radiation, five days a week for five weeks, will follow about a month later.

As my main job now is to get as strong as possible before surgery, Larry and I have decided to go to Mexico in February, where we will spend a few days in Oaxaca and then a couple of weeks on the

Pacific coast. I'm hoping it will be pure R&R, and that I'll come home stronger, resilient, and ready to face the next steps on this journey.

So many of you sent cards, e-mails, letters, and healing gifts and delivered delicious meals following my dad's death. Please know how much these thoughtful gestures mean to me. Let's hope 2010 is a better year for all of us.

Be well. Carpe diem.
Love, Tamara

Reflections

MOURNING MY FATHER

My dad's death left a huge hole in my heart and in my life. I walked around in a daze, sleeping fitfully, exhausted and spent. My tears flowed freely and often, spurred on by any association with Dad. I wondered, is this what grief is? I had known grief, had lived inside it following my diagnosis. But it had plunged to new depths.

Two friends organized a non-traditional shiva on a Sunday afternoon a few days before my next round of chemo. As we gathered to remember my dad with the November sun pouring through the windows into pools of light on the floor, we went around the circle sharing memories with photographs, stories, and songs. My mom sang "Lula Lula Bye Bye," a lullaby Paul Robeson had sung. Ellen "recited" the Shema prayer in graceful, dance-like sign language. Joni and Tunde played their haunting guitars as the rest of us sang along. Afterwards my tears still flowed, but I felt newly embraced, grateful to have honored my father and my grief this way, appreciating how essential to my mourning this observance had been.

A couple of weeks later, I was pleased to hear that Rachel had also had her own version of a shiva in Montreal. Although many of her friends weren't Jewish and hadn't known her grandfather, Rachel invited them to her apartment to share memories, look at pictures, play some of the music he'd loved, and eat some of his favorite foods together.

Karen, my mom, Larry, and I now had to plan the more public memorial, knowing it would be a mammoth undertaking. I worried about how my mom was doing living on her own for the first time, grieving while trying to cope with the mountains of paperwork a death inevitably requires. We had to get copies of his death certificate, see the estate lawyer, deal with Dad's will, and search his filing cabinet for documents. We had to cancel his passport, driver's license, credit cards, and everything else that was in his name, change all the billing to my mom's name, and dispose of his car. At the same time, I was preparing to start on Taxotere. In the midst of mourning, I had to find a way to carry on with treatment and my life.

TAXOTERE: THE MACK TRUCK OF CHEMO

At my support group, some of the women had already experienced the ravages of Taxotere. Marta and Claudia described ending up in hospital. Their resistance was so low that infections had set in following their chemo sessions. Marta, a diminutive and expressive woman from Mexico, waved her hands in the air and clutched her belly as she described her agony.

How could I prepare myself for what loomed ahead as the "Mack truck" of chemo? It felt like I was getting ready to be hit by a train.

What about my white blood cell count? I was relieved when Dr. Verma prescribed pegfilgrastim (Neulasta) and that our drug plans would cover it. Claudia had not been asked whether she had a drug plan. She hadn't known about the possibility of receiving Neulasta because her doctor hadn't told her about it. Even though it might have helped fight her cancer, she had decided to stop Taxotere after the first round because it had completely traumatized her. Ironically, her time in emergency and her stay in hospital cost the health care system far more than what Neulasta would have cost. Claudia told me she and her husband would have found a way to pay for the Neulasta if they had been told about it.

Claudia's experience drove home a major problem in the cancer care system. You, the patient, are utterly dependent on your own particular oncologist (or surgeon) to find out about a critical treatment or preventive therapy that can make an enormous difference to your health and well-being. There is too much inconsistency between the specialists, the knowledge and information they have, and what they can or are willing to offer their patients. This inevitably has a negative impact on standards of care. One of the most valuable aspects of being part of the support group was being able to share both our positive and negative experiences. Stories like Claudia's and Marta's propelled me to find out if there was anything out there to help avoid what they had gone through. None of us should have to be guinea pigs, especially when there are known solutions.

I had done everything I could with both Leesa and Dr. Verma to prepare for Taxotere. I was relieved that they had spoken to each other and worked out a plan. Now I had to prepare myself psychologically and spiritually to receive it, to find a way to welcome the toxic brew into my body to fight my cancer and receive the drug's healing powers. At the same time, I knew it could break me.

In the past, I'd had a pretty high pain threshold. I'd given birth without epidurals or anesthetics. I preferred to have little or no freezing at the dentist's office. I hardly ever had headaches or took painkillers. But I knew this pain would be different from anything I had experienced before.

My heart was in my mouth as Larry and I arrived at the chemo room. I had been in a reclining chair for my first four rounds of chemo, but this time the nurse had me lie down on a bed, propped up my head with pillows and a put a heated flannel blanket over me. I shivered when she put large mitts that looked like oven mitts filled with ice on my hands and ice slippers on my feet. She told me they would help keep my finger and toe nails from breaking and help prevent neuropathy, numbness in my hands and feet. The nurse watched me like a hawk, checking my pulse, taking my temperature, asking me how I was doing. Other than the pain from the cold that made my hands and feet feel like ice blocks about to break off from my body, I managed to get through my first round of Taxotere without incident. But I knew the worst was yet to come.

I had already ordered the shot of Neulasta from the pharmacy, picking up the precious ampoule of liquid gold on the day after chemo. The home care nurse arrived that afternoon. She sat down on the couch beside me as she cleaned my upper right arm with alcohol. I looked straight ahead as she positioned the needle carefully before pushing the plunger of the syringe and injecting its contents into my arm. Larry watched carefully as he studied her moves, knowing he would be the one to give me the shots later on. I felt strangely "lucky," relieved to know the injection might keep me stable and out of hospital.

I didn't feel at all well, but I managed until Day 6. Then the Mack truck arrived in full force, blasting through my lower body, crushing the bones in my pelvis and legs like a bulldozer on a rampage. I felt as if my bones were becoming liquid, rubbery, dissolving into molten lava on the inside. I could hardly stand up. My tears poured out unceasingly, blurring my vision and crusting my face with salt as I tried to mop them up. I couldn't see well enough to read the newspaper below the headlines. I'd taken virtually no painkillers until that point, but now I swallowed a couple and headed for bed, praying for sleep. Wake me when it's over.

I crawled out of bed a little later, unable to sleep, clutching myself, feeling queasy and wretched. When my mom arrived at the house that night, I could barely speak. I knew she could hardly stand to see me in pain, but as she had so many times since I'd been diagnosed, she rose valiantly to take care of me. She asked if I wanted my head rubbed. I lay down on the couch, curled up in fetal position, my bald head resting on a pillow in her lap. Larry brought a soft blanket to cover me. My mom stroked me for hours, her practiced hands gentle, her voice soothing. Afterwards, I hugged her as she went out the door, watching her clutch the wooden railing as she descended the porch stairs into the cold night. At eighty-six she was old, but that night I was the frail one. I held on to the banister as I began my slow climb upstairs to my bed.

I found out later that Taxotere attacks the bone marrow, which explains why my bones felt like they were liquefying from the inside. I also learned that when chemo attacks cells, it zeroes in on where we are most vulnerable. My eyes became an open target, which meant there would be times when I was seriously visually impaired. For Gwen in my support group, it was her hip. Her hip had been weak for a few years, but it became increasingly painful and debilitated as she progressed through chemo. She was set to have it replaced when she finished her last round.

The good news was that when I saw Dr. Verma just before my sixth round of chemo, he could feel that my tumors had already shrunk significantly. When I told him about my Mack truck experience, he prescribed extra doses of an antidote. There was nothing he could do for my eyes. Taxotere was a hell of a drug, but it was working.

STRADDLING CHALLENGES

Since the chemo was working and my tumors were shrinking, I could now start on intravenous vitamin C.

I believe that the support I was getting from Leesa, was doing yeoman's duty to complement the medical care I was getting from the Cancer Centre. Combined with healthy food and exercise, I was doing what I could to get well. It reinforced how my decision to straddle mainstream and complementary medicine made sense for me. One of my challenges had been to find out whether Dr. Verma was open to the idea of my working with Leesa.

Leesa explained how intravenous vitamin C acts like natural chemotherapy. Known for years to offer protection against cancer, it protects cellular structures from damage and helps the body deal with environmental pollution and toxic chemicals. It boosts the immune function and inhibits cancer-causing compounds from forming. Recently, scientific evidence is showing that vitamin C preferentially kills cancer cells, meaning it is only toxic to cancer cells and not to normal healthy cells. For vitamin C to work this way, it must be given in high doses of 50 to 100 grams. There is a limit to the amount of vitamin C that can be absorbed orally. However, when higher doses are administered intravenously and the digestive system is by-passed, cancer cells are killed and other cells remain unharmed.

When I first met Dr. Verma, I was already working with Leesa, taking naturopathic supplements and planning to see her for acupuncture before and after each chemo session. I told Dr. Verma about Leesa's practice, described her proposal for how she would work with me and gave him a list of my supplements. I was relieved when he said he didn't have a problem with my taking the supplements.

Reassured, I decided to take the next step. Leesa had told me that if I could receive vitamin C intravenously two or three times a week throughout my four rounds of Taxotere, it would maximize the effectiveness of the chemo and lessen its side effects. It made sense, but I knew I wasn't ready to go ahead without Dr. Verma's blessing. I didn't know if he'd be open to the idea, but the next time I saw him, I asked if he'd be willing to talk to Leesa on the phone to discuss their respective approaches to my situation. I especially wanted them to discuss the possibility of receiving intravenous vitamin C (IVC) during the upcoming chemo.

Leesa and Dr. Verma came up with a protocol. I would go through my first round without the IVC to make sure the chemo was working, which Dr. Verma would determine when he checked whether my tumors were shrinking. If it was working, I would receive IVC during the two non-chemo weeks between each of my last three rounds. I was overjoyed when Leesa told me that she and Dr.

Dr. Shailendra Verma: You can't come from my culture and not respect what complementary approaches have to offer. When I was 13, I developed acne. I was terribly ashamed of this. Every doctor I saw, dermatologists, etc. tried to treat me. But the person who helped me most was a homeopathic doctor, and within two weeks I was fine. So I had an experience that altered my own life.

Verma had had a good conversation. She was pleased to have taken the first step toward establishing a respectful working relationship with such an esteemed oncologist. She hoped it might help pave the way for other doctors to support their patients who wanted to work with naturopaths.

Although I was relieved, I also knew I had to be careful about whether, when, how, and to whom I talked about my forays into complementary medicine. I was aware that for many breast cancer patients, this was a strange and mysterious new world. For example, I sensed it would have been too much for some of the women in my support group to consider another layer of treatment on top of what they were already coping with. Some were interested in exploring alternative approaches, and had bravely broached the possibility with their oncologists and surgeons. Too often, they met with rolling eyes and disparaging comments. Understandably, some of them were then too fearful to venture into territory that might alienate the doctors they felt their lives depended on at a time when they felt so vulnerable. (Of course, there are plenty of unregulated quacks out there willing to prey on sick, desperate people for profit, but I'm talking about licensed bona fide naturopaths.)

Dr. Joanne Meng: I don't know a lot about the field. I'm not opposed to it nor do I know how to embrace it. But having talked to Leesa and after working with you, I don't feel animosity or resistance. I'm completely open to learning more about it.

Dr. Angel Arnaout: I fully support complementary cancer care. None of us have all the answers: we certainly are not able to treat 100 percent of our patients effectively.

Dr. Shailendra Verma: As oncologists, we need to change our approach to complementary care. Thankfully, the newer stream of oncologists is more receptive. It will take an attitude shift. People who want complementary cancer care need to say, "It's my cancer. I need to get better. These are the routes that I need to get better with." End of story.

There is also the question of cost. Although the price of most forms of complementary care is far less than traditional medicine, it is expensive to the individual patient because public health care funding does not cover it. Few extended health plans give more than nominal support for complementary medicine. This means that those who seek it out need to have enough resources to pay the cost or be willing to go into debt at a time when their income is already drastically reduced. In Canada, the price of chemo, surgery, and radiation to treat one woman's breast cancer is about $50,000. The cost of naturopathic treatment for the same cancer is a small fraction of that amount, between $5,000 and $10,000.

Another issue is that there has been less money to carry out extensive (and expensive) clinical trials on complementary therapies. The evidence produced by these trials is the accepted foundation of medical treatment. Generally underwritten by large pharmaceutical companies, there is tremendous profit to be made once the drugs are shown to be safe and effective and are approved by governments. But complementary medicine uses products from natural sources that can't be patented. Most governments have been unwilling to support clinical trials on such products, and there is no financial incentive for drug companies to fund the research.

> **Dr. Leesa Kirchner:** Part of the draw for me to join the Integrative Cancer Centre was that more people will know about complementary care. Hopefully, more people will be able to afford it too. Our services are a bit cheaper because we're non-profit and we have a sliding scale so more people can access and afford this kind of care.

There are, however, other valid forms of evidence that show the value and effectiveness of various therapies used within complementary medicine for cancer care. While clinical trials for therapies such as vitamin D and intravenous vitamin C are starting on a small scale, there is still a long way to go. In an ideal world, naturopaths, homeopaths, acupuncturists, and other complementary therapists would

Dr. Shailendra Verma: For too long, disciplines have worked in isolation without communication and our patients have felt caught between differing therapeutic philosophies, often to their detriment. An integrative program will provide a much needed bridge.

work alongside medical doctors in hospitals, clinics, and other cancer care centers, and the costs of both research and delivery would be covered by public health care funds.

GENETIC TESTING

I was stunned when Dr. Verma asked me during our first appointment if I was an Ashkenazi Jew, and that he went on to recommend genetic testing when I said I was. Going through genetic testing was loaded with anxiety because of the litany of horrors that could be triggered by the results of the blood test. It began with a meeting with a genetic counselor. She compassionately but straightforwardly explained what is known about breast cancer and the percentages of cases that are linked to hereditary (15 to 20 percent) versus environmental causes or that are simply sporadic. She then went through my family tree, dredging up all I knew of the medical histories of my grandparents, their siblings and offspring. She invited the genetic oncologist to go over the implications for both me and my kids if the tests determined I was carrying the mutated gene.

We discussed whether Larry might be a carrier given the history of breast cancer in his mother's family. At our appointment, Dr. Verma had urged Larry to be tested, as both men and women of Ashkanazi descent are four times more likely to carry the gene than the general population, although men rarely develop breast cancer. Dr. Verma's words to Larry were "spare her," referring to Rachel, because if both of us were negative, she wouldn't have to worry that she'd inherited the gene. If one or both of us were positive, she could either choose to have the genetic test herself or opt for rigorous monitoring starting at age thirty or so.

With what felt like the weight of the world on my shoulders, I figured I had little choice. There was a 22 percent chance I was a carrier. If I was a carrier, there was an 80 percent chance that my breast cancer would recur. I figured I might as well know about it so I could do what I could to keep it from coming back. The test would determine whether I had any of the three mutations most common in the Ashkenazi population (out of about 700 possible mutations overall).

My die was cast. For me, it wasn't a question of knowing whether I'd get breast cancer because I already had it. Rather, it was about harm reduction, of doing what was possible to improve my chances for a longer and better quality of life. I was sick at the prospect of my body being butchered by even more invasive surgery and of the elevated risk of a recurrence. But I was more anguished that the results could reveal the corollary knowledge that I might have unwittingly passed the deadly gene to one or both of my children. What would such an ominous piece of information mean for how they lived their lives?

FACING MY OWN MORTALITY

I never imagined I'd be staring the Grim Reaper in the face at fifty-eight. But here I was, diagnosed with a highly aggressive breast cancer. The possibility of an early death became suddenly real and palpable. No one ever explicitly said "You could die from this," or "You should get your affairs in order." But I had an aggressive Stage III, Grade 3, locally advanced triple negative breast cancer.

I knew that no one dies from breast cancer, that it is fatal only when it travels to other parts of the body. Because my cancer had already spread from my breast to my lymph nodes, there was no way of knowing if it had also traveled farther afield. The possibility of dying loomed large for the first time in my life. It was hard to imagine no longer being in the world, being extinguished, leaving my family behind, not having the chance to get old, not being able to do so many of the things I still wanted to do. I not only feared death itself but also what the getting there would be like, the unspeakable pain and suffering that comes before death, the often prolonged and torturous process of dying for those with terminal cancer.

During the first few weeks following my diagnosis, death became my constant, uninvited companion, my shadow, always present although not always apparent. It was with me every hour of the day and night, hovering, no matter what I was doing. I could be at home or elsewhere, alone or with others. I would get caught up in something and forget it momentarily, but then it would nudge me, whisper in my ear, or subtly put the weight of its hand on my shoulder. I would take a deep breath, register its presence and acknowledge its undeniable power and eminence.

I hadn't chosen to become better acquainted with death. But since there was a chance I wouldn't make it, I needed to consider what dying would look like. I imagined the painful good-byes, the losses on all sides. I'd conjure up what my life would look like without me in it and watch the grainy film as the reels played out, my blank silhouette in every frame.

I figured that the only way I was going to have the courage to fight this cancer was to bring death front and center into my consciousness and accept that it was now a part of me. Once it was firmly planted, I could stare it down, reckon and banter with it, even try to make deals with it. As death gradually became more familiar, it struck me that my dread was lessening. I became increasingly fearless as it started to lift. I thought if I had both wrestled with and befriended death, what was there left to fear? When I read Audre Lorde's *The Cancer Journals* (1980) about the celebrated poet's experience with breast cancer, her words spoke eloquently: "What is there possibly left for us to be afraid of, after we have dealt face to face with death and not embraced it? Once I accept the existence of dying as a life process, who can ever have power over me again?"

I carried my new relationship with death forward into other situations. The first was the experience of my dad's death. As we watched him fade, I dreaded the prospect of losing him. But at the same time, I had a growing familiarity with death as the visitor in our midst and its place at the table in our lives. In my first letter to my mom, I wrote: "Now I stare my mortality in the face, as it is possible that this cancer will kill me. Thinking, ironically, that this mortality thing is something we now have in common at this point in our lives."

Later, several fellow cancer patients in Leesa's vitamin C room died during the time I was going for regular treatments. As difficult as it was to cope with the losses of people I had come to care about, I needed to know when one had died. Their deaths were a part of life, part of the experience of cancer, and part of our collective story.

We can't grow up in North America without developing illusions and fears about death, no matter what our religious or cultural background. Separated from the inherent naturalness of death, we have a vocabulary that denies or makes fun of death at the same time as we lack a common language for naming and talking honestly about the conclusion of our life cycle. We keep people with no chance of recovery alive on life support while we deny effective pain management and good palliative care to those who are suffering. If we are so collectively inept at dealing with death, what do we do when its harbinger arrives unannounced and uninvited at our doorstep?

It is useful to become familiar with the prospect of our deaths in our own way. There is no right or wrong way to do this, and each of us must find our path to get there. If we can find a way to confront

Joyce Hardman: When you start to get an inkling of the grayness of life, something starts to shift and your toleration for the unknown opens up a little. Somebody dies, and you discover that there is no trustworthy permanent situation and that life just keeps on changing. Ultimately, you come to a place where you say "I can do the best I can with now, I can be as conscious as I can with now. I have no guarantee what will happen next, but I'm willing to walk into it."

our darkest fears, including our fear of dying, we will be less afraid. We will be stronger in our resolve to live each day as fully as possible while we fight our cancers or any other life-threatening illness with everything we have.

CHAPTER SIX

Finishing Chemo
and Detoxing in Mexico

As my eighth and last round of chemotherapy approached, I could hardly believe the first leg of my journey through treatment was almost over. In my mind, I had ranked the various treatments as a descending hierarchy of evils. I saw chemotherapy as the worst offender, followed by surgery, and then radiation as the least of the ordeals. Of course, I had only experienced chemo, but I imagined I'd be through the worst of it when I was done.

I had survived my first seven rounds. The experience had been lousy, even horrible at times. But after a while, I'd learned to roll with the rhythm of my three-week cycles. I braced myself for the blackout days that followed each treatment. I looked forward to the waning of my queasiness and later of my "liquid bones" as the heaviness dissipated. I rejoiced when my energy and sense of well-being started to return for most of my second and third weeks, when I'd "max out" on doing the things I yearned to do. Then, just as I was feeling at my relative best, I'd prepare to get knocked down again.

I knew the shape and structure of my life would change again once chemo was over. Vast, uncharted territory lay ahead. I would lose some of the good things that had become part of my everyday life. My sister would no longer be spending weekends with me. The Supper Sisters wouldn't be bringing us meals as regularly. I wouldn't be visiting Dr. Verma as often to see how I was doing and confirm that my tumors were shrinking.

Most importantly, my cancer wouldn't be under the constant attack it had been through over the past several months. I couldn't help but wonder if there were still errant cancer cells lurking within me. If chemo isn't on their case 24/7, will this be their chance to escape? Thankfully, I would continue to work with Leesa, receiving intravenous vitamin C and taking supplements to strengthen my immune system and fight off any lingering cancer cells.

On the other hand, the brutal treatments would be over. My battered body could finally start on its long journey to reclaim itself. It could begin to heal. Maybe my hair would even start to grow back! Larry and I had the crazy idea of going to Mexico for three weeks between the end of chemo and my surgery. We bought tickets to leave for Oaxaca twelve days after my last chemo. We hoped it would be a time for healing.

✉ Healing Journey #6

March 7, 2010

Dear friends and family,

I approached my last round of chemo on January 28th with both trepidation about the impending side effects and relief that it would soon be over. There was no doubt that Missy's offer to come back and sing me through my last round of chemo made it more palatable.

When I saw Dr. Verma a couple of days earlier, he was pleased with how well the chemo was working as my tumors appeared to have shrunk by more than 50 percent. We hoped this would be confirmed by an MRI a few days hence. After the appointment, I went to the chemo room to make sure it was okay to bring Missy to sing when I returned for my treatment. I was stunned when the head nurse told me there had been a complaint the last time, and that if Missy came she could only sing a couple of songs.

I was devastated. I couldn't understand how anyone could have complained. The patients, their families, and the nurses had all seemed to enjoy the music, tapping their feet and making requests. Jim, an elderly patient, even attributed the drop in his blood pressure to the music. The only reason I could think of for anyone to complain was that they had been assigned to a different pod and had felt left out!

Now, not only would chemo be more difficult without the singing as it dripped into my veins for the last time, but I would have to find a way to tell Missy. Thankfully, she had a thicker skin than I. She helped me see that some people on chemo may not appreciate our spirited singing because of what they are dealing with. She said she wanted to come to my last round anyway.

Larry and I picked Missy up the next morning, leaving her guitar in the car in the hospital parking lot. The nurse who was setting me up in the bed was especially friendly, so we decided to tell her what had happened to our plan to sing. She came up with the brilliant idea to ask the head nurse if we could use the empty isolation room across the hall reserved for seriously ill patients. Happily, the head nurse gave us her blessing. We retrieved the guitar and moved to the private room.

In the end, we sang and told stories through my last chemo just as we had hoped. Maybe it was even better because we had turned lemons into lemonade, and the nurses who came in to take care of me sang along with us. On our way out, Larry, Missy, and I each took a turn pulling the yellow ribbon that rings the cast iron bell on the wall. Everyone around us cheered, a long-standing tradition as patients finish their last round of chemo, hoping never to return. Hallelujah!

The first three post-chemo days were a whirlwind of activity. Larry and I went to a pre-surgery information session at Breast Cancer Action. I went for acupuncture with my naturopath, saw my chiropractor, baked bread for the first time, worked out at the Y, had a manicure and pedicure, and sang with the band for the Tu B'shvat holiday.

That last infusion of chemo, however, didn't let me down easily. Exhaustion hit on Day 4, and I spent the day collapsed on my bed. To add insult to injury, a nasty infection set in above my upper lip and was swelling, oozing, and crusting over, making it look like I'd been kicked in the mouth. I was especially discouraged about my eyes, which were watering like fountains, blurring my vision, and getting in the way of reading and driving. As my lip (now diagnosed as a staph infection and treated with antibiotic cream) and eye problems continued, I started to worry about whether I'd be able to chair or even attend the upcoming Inter Pares board meeting. Would I be in any shape to leave on our trip to Mexico a few days later? What had I been thinking?

On Day 8, although I was still feeling and looking rotten, I went ahead with plans to go shopping with Ellen for head gear for Mexico. Thankfully she drove, as my vision was so blurred I could hardly distinguish between the colors of the traffic lights. We headed to Freda's, the hair salon and wig store in a nondescript strip mall where I had bought my wig and had my head tenderly shaved almost five months earlier. The hairdresser, who on my first visits had been so kind and patient, remembered me and happily showed us her assortment of head gear. After buying a couple of caps, she suggested we go next door to see what Kelly's Mastectomy Shop had to offer.

I knew Kelly's carried prostheses, bras and bathing suits for women who had gone through mastectomies, but I wasn't prepared for the array of fashion in the store. Once again, the staff were attentive, nonplussed by my bald head, and appearing to have all the time in the world as we tried on hats and scarves. At the cash, I asked the owner who Kelly was. She pointed to a large photograph on the wall of her brother's wife, Kelly, who had died of breast cancer a few years earlier at thirty-two, leaving a young daughter. She started and carries on the business in honor of Kelly.

Over a Lebanese lunch in the strip mall, Ellen and I marveled at the amazing women who run and work at these businesses. Without fanfare, these unsung heroines have created sanctuaries for women dealing with cancer.

A couple of days later, I received a voice mail message from my "angel" surgeon, Dr. Angel Arnaout, who had the results of my post-chemo MRI. There appeared to be no evidence of cancer on the MRI, which meant the chemo plus the complementary therapies had worked! She would still need to go ahead with the lumpectomy and removal of my lymph nodes to make sure there were clean margins around where the tumors had been, but she was very pleased. I listened to the message several times before it sunk in. While I was feeling too wrecked to be ecstatic, I was hugely relieved.

Two days later, heeding the advice of my mother and sister to book wheelchairs for the Toronto and Mexico City airports, Larry and I got on a plane to Oaxaca in the wee dark hours of the morning of February 9th.

We knew this would be a holiday like no other. I wasn't really thinking of it as a holiday, but rather as a "detox" from the chemicals that had been running through my body since starting chemo. It would also be a chance to get as strong as possible for my surgery to take place on March 9th, a week after our return. We agreed to take it easy in Mexico and to pace ourselves accordingly.

We loved staying at a homey B&B in Oaxaca where we had a great time over the fabulous Mexican breakfasts sharing stories with the cast of characters there, including three feisty forty-something women from Toronto. In the mornings after breakfast, Larry and I ventured out into this beautiful colonial city, rich in history and culture, returning to rest in the hammock or around the pool in the afternoons. While this normally would have been prime time for reading, my eyes continued to plague me as they watered and blurred excessively, leaving me frustrated, discouraged, and unable to read.

We had a magical night on Valentine's (*El Día del Amor*) eve, *la Noce de las Luces*, wandering the streets of Oaxaca. The air was balmy and electric. Oaxacenos of every age were on the streets walking arm in arm: families with grandparents and young children, lovers, vendors with giant bouquets of red heart-shaped balloons, everyone greeting each other. Music was everywhere: a singing guitar orchestra outside a church, kids folk dancing in traditional costumes on a makeshift stage in the street, a candlelight parade to the *Zocolo* in the center of the city, fireworks. I thought about how different it was from Valentine's Day in Canada in the middle of winter, usually a private affair of cards, flowers, and chocolate. In Mexico, it isn't just about romantic love but about *amor y amistad*, love and friendship, which seems to be a more inclusive way to celebrate.

We were invited for supper with the Gomez family thanks to a mutual Mexican friend in Ottawa, Luz Maria. While I was looking forward to meeting the family, I was worried about my limited stamina and didn't want to insult them if I had to leave early by Mexican standards because of my health. I decided to call ahead to say it would need to be an early evening for me because I had breast cancer and was recovering from chemo. Shortly afterwards, the family arrived at our B&B bearing a Valentine gift, deeply concerned, wondering how they could help. I assured them I wasn't in crisis. I just wanted to let them know about my situation and say how much we were looking forward to spending time with them. Later that evening, they welcomed us as we drank wine on their roof garden and enjoyed a delicious Oaxacan supper in English, Spanish, and translation. In spite of the language barrier, I believe we were able to openly share the ups and downs of our lives at a deeper level because the emotional floodgates had opened.

We had planned to spend the next two weeks in Puerto Escondido on the Pacific coast, but saw almost immediately that it would be an enormous challenge for me. Although our B&B there was an oasis of tranquility with a small pool, it was a long walk to the 140 steps going down to the closest beach. So when our Toronto friends told us about their cabana in a small fishing village on a pristine beach down the coast, we decided to head south for our last week.

San Augustinillo had been at the heart of the turtle industry and home to a processing plant for turtle meat, long considered a delicacy. In 1990, the Mexican government declared sea turtles endangered, made fishing them illegal, and is now trying to develop eco-tourism in the area. We fell in love with the village, our cabana, and the beach.

I was getting stronger by the day, taking long walks on the beach, listening to the surf, drinking in the brilliant sunsets. I had two major breakthroughs soon after our arrival. First, I ventured into the ocean in my bathing cap and goggles, where I joyously swam and played in the waves. Then, in the small library where we were staying, I found a book printed in a large font, which meant I could spend glorious hours in the hammock, reading happily.

We swam, walked, played Upwords; had delicious meals with new friends from Toronto, South Africa, and Denmark; and paddled through a lagoon of mangroves with iguanas, turtles, and crocodiles.

On a hike, we encountered a funky wedding party where the couple said their vows against the backdrop of a magnificent sunset and the full moon rising over the majestic Punta Cometa. I even braved going out in a fishing boat early one morning. Thankfully, the sea was calm so I didn't get sick, and it was thrilling to see birds, dolphins, sea turtles, and a mother whale with her babe so close up. While it was sad to leave San Augustinillo, I left rejuvenated. I was as strong and ready as I could be to face my impending surgery. I also knew we would be back.

It's strange, anticipating surgery and the prospect of being cut in such tender and sensitive areas of my body, anticipating pain. I think I'm probably more fearful of the lymph node dissection in my underarm than I am of the lumpectomy, although I know it would be different if I were facing a mastectomy. But lymph node dissection is an invasive surgery that removes a large chunk of flesh, resulting in a weakened lymphatic system. It's also part of a critical joint in the shoulder and underarm that is key to movement in many directions.

Although the procedure is usually day surgery, my surgeon told me she will keep me overnight at the hospital because I've been on chemo and she wants to give me as much support as possible. I'm grateful for that, although I know I'll also be more susceptible to infection in the hospital.

I'll go home the next day. I'll be bandaged for several days with a drain in my underarm and pills for the pain. I'll need to wear tops with buttons down the front for a while as I won't be able to lift my arms over my head to put on T-shirts or turtlenecks. I can't have a full shower for ten days. I'm supposed to start doing exercises right away to avoid lymphedema, the swelling of the arm due to a compromised lymphatic system. Larry will be with me, my mom and Daniel too, and Karen will arrive from Toronto and Rachel from Montreal. Joyce, my coach, will come over to help me meditate.

Joyce Hardman: Often people start meditating at this time. Meditation is a practice of helplessness in a way because it's a practice of not trying to change anything, but of just being still, just sitting there in the mystery.

It will be tough. I loathe having to give up my newfound strength and sense of well-being that has been with me for such a short time. I dread the pain and having less mobility in my arm. At the same time, I know I have a skilled and caring surgeon, and that the lumpectomy will be less invasive because of the positive results of the MRI. My naturopath has put me on a homeopathic regimen to minimize pain and to promote healing. I have done, I think, what I can do to prepare myself.

Tomorrow, March 8th, is International Women's Day. It is a time to celebrate the incredible gains of the women's movement, and to reflect on where to go from here. There is still so much inequality, violence, and lack of education for girls and women all over the world, still so much more to be done. For me, it is also a time to appreciate sisterhood and the many women who have been there for me in so many ways since this journey began. There have also been some wonderful men in my life.

So many of you have sent your good wishes with the hope that my surgery will go well. They are so much appreciated, and I will go under knowing that you are with me, sending your healing energy.

Be well. Carpe diem.
Love, Tamara

Reflections

PUTTING THE "TEAM" TOGETHER

I was grateful to have Leesa and Dr. Verma on my team and collabo-
rating on a protocol that allowed me to receive intravenous vitamin
C during chemo. But the team wasn't complete yet: I'd asked around
for names of a good surgeon because I couldn't bear the thought of
going under a knife held by the first surgeon I'd met. The hospital had
referred me to Dr. Joanne Meng, a radiation oncologist whom I liked
immediately for her warmth and straight talking manner. Although
radiation wouldn't be happening for several months, it was good to
meet her and to feel confident about the doctor who would be in
charge of that phase. I held my breath as I dared ask Dr. Meng if she
could make a referral on my behalf to Dr. Angel Arnaout, a highly
regarded breast cancer surgeon I'd heard about. Dr. Meng agreed to
see what she could do, and a couple of weeks later, I had an appointment with Dr. Arnaout. It seemed like a miracle that my "team" was
coming together!

FOR WHOM THE BELL TOLLS

When I heard there had been a complaint about Missy's singing, I was
stunned and disappointed. The music had been such a comforting
balm to me as well as to several other patients. The thought of going
through my last round without Missy while surrounded by the bad
karma of the complaint felt depressing, even ominous.

I didn't know how to tell Missy and worried she'd be offended or
hurt. But Missy was a former nurse who knew hospital politics well
and understood how complaints are handled with kid gloves. When
I told her, she threw her head back, groaned loudly, and laughed. She
insisted on coming along anyway.

But the incident made me think hard about how my experience

might be different from that of other patients, including the anonymous complainer. Other patients might be living with terrible pain. Or they might be receiving palliative chemo to try to alleviate their symptoms or prolong their lives for a few more weeks. They might be alone or upset, or their families might be falling apart. It's possible that any sound, even lovely music, was irritating or unnerving, and thus unwanted.

For me, the music was about hope. I was hungry for it and couldn't get enough of it. Music had always got me through hard times and times of sorrow. Although I badly wanted the singing, I could now see how it was presumptuous of me to assume anything about anyone else's situation and whether they would want or appreciate the music. I had to respect where they were coming from, even if it flew in the face of what I wanted.

Once we landed in the bizarre sanctuary of the isolation room, we sang our hearts out, the music stirring up deep wells of both sadness and relief within me. A couple of hours later when the last drops of chemo were gone and they unhooked me from the IV one last time, I was thrilled but utterly spent.

Liberated at last, it was time for Larry, Missy, and me to walk arm in arm down the hallway to ring the chemo bell. I hadn't thought much about who gets to ring the chemo bell before I rang it. It had seemed like a hopeful and fitting goal to aspire to, a ritual to mark the end of chemo, celebrate that I had run the gauntlet of this phase of treatment and rejoice because the chemo had worked. I felt triumphant as we took turns pulling the long yellow ribbon attached to the school bell, its ring reverberating down the hall as the patients and nurses cheered us on from the sidelines. Of course, I imagined it would be the same for the other patients.

It was only later that I thought about the others, the patients who might never get to ring the bell. Those were patients whose cancers would never be in remission, who might never be well again, who could end up on chemo for the rest of their lives, however long that was to be. What was it like for them to see folks like me jubilantly ringing the bell? It was as if, at least for now, I was being let out of a prison from which they would never be liberated. It was yet another reminder that, as cancer patients, our health, good fortune, and hope for the future are both relative and precarious.

CUMULATIVE EFFECT

The effects of chemo are cumulative, so I knew this last round would hit the hardest. It would also boost the combined healing power of all the treatments I'd received to date. I came crashing down with a vengeance a couple of days after the last round, sicker and weaker than I had been after any other session. I felt wobbly and depleted, a sorry and wasted bag of bones. The worst part was my eyes. I'd always had one good and one weak eye, and I'd had surgery on my weak eye as a young child. My good eye had always done almost all the work. A year earlier, I had developed a cataract on my good eye, but so far it hadn't been considered "ripe" enough for surgery.

Now I was always mopping up the tears that filled up my eyes and streamed down my face, blurring my vision. I knew it would have been unsafe to drive, although I didn't feel much like driving anyway. What devastated me was that I couldn't even read the newspaper beyond the headlines. I had managed to get through the difficult days as long as I could read and write, but when these were gone I was beside myself.

To add insult to injury, I had a nasty infection above my upper lip. There I was in all my glory, a weak, bald, browless creature with pale, sallow skin. I was practically blind, watering from my eyes, and sporting a gross and unsightly upper lip. I had reached a new low that was worse than being raw and unvarnished. Now I was ugly, miserable, and visually impaired. When I was brave enough to glance in the mirror, I saw a sick, withered old woman I barely recognized. My only consolation was that I couldn't see well enough to know how bad I really looked!

I had had trouble coping with the loss of feeling at all attractive since the early days of chemo. But now, the loss of my former physical self was scaling new heights. Most days, I wore one of my standard, understated "uniforms:" a turtleneck, vest, and pants with a bandana or my wig. My only concession to adornment was to wear long scarves and my trademark large hoop earrings, without which I felt completely naked. Even this incidental nod to fashion was minimalist. Although I had dozens of earrings, I wore the same couple of pairs. I had never been a big shopper, but on the few occasions when I'd gone into stores since starting treatment, I shunned mirrors and dressing rooms. I didn't mind scouting the racks for my sister or a friend, but I had no interest in shopping for myself. I refused to try anything on because it would have involved exposing and then adorning myself, efforts in futility doomed to bring on even more dejection.

MAGICAL THINKING IN MEXICO

Larry and I had come up with the idea of going to Mexico sometime in the fall during chemo, probably in one of my better weeks when such a trip seemed possible. Taking a break between chemo and surgery made sense, especially since the hiatus would take place during the dead of winter.

Our thinking was that the warm air, sun, and ocean would do us good. Larry loved leaving winter behind to get the fix of sun he craved. I looked forward to giving my body a chance to detox and begin to heal. It would be a break from "the cancer bubble," as Larry called it. I knew I couldn't leave cancer behind me, but I was up for a change of scene. It would also be a way to have some solid time together away and to reconnect as we usually did on holidays. It might even bring a bit of magic back into our lives.

But Mexico might as well have been Mars at that point. What

could Larry and I have been thinking when we had planned our trip? It was an act of magical thinking to imagine we could pull it off. Leaving twelve days after my last chemo had seemed reasonable enough at the time we booked our flights based on my previous chemo experiences. We had agreed to take it slowly and easily once we got there, but after being struck down by my last chemo blow, the whole idea seemed ludicrous. It was complicated because we hadn't planned a predictable package holiday, but had booked flights and made reservations for a few days each at in Oaxaca and Puerto Escondido. We planned to play the rest by ear. We hadn't even bought cancellation insurance.

Luz Maria had lots of suggestions and was helpful and encouraging when I had asked her about visiting Oaxaca. But she called a few days later to tell me about a conversation she'd had with a doctor friend in Mexico. She said she felt badly, but had to pass along his somber warning that I would be unwise to travel to Mexico in my current state. He'd said, "You never know what kind of reaction you might have to a new environment when your immune system is compromised after chemo." I swallowed the advice hard, then carried on as if we were going to Mexico anyway, hoping my strength would rally in time.

I hadn't thought about going to a travel medicine clinic before the trip. After all, I'd been to Mexico many times before, and had never worried about getting shots. Now flattened by my last chemo session, I realized that as a cancer patient, my situation was different. Also, we were going to a part of the country where I had never traveled.

When I finally called the travel medicine clinic, the doctor was away, so I didn't get to see him until a couple of days before our departure. I guess I shouldn't have been surprised when, after he heard I'd just finished chemo, he wanted me to have my white blood cell count tested. He called me the same day with my test results. He said that my cell count was high, indicating that I likely had an infection, and strongly advised me to delay the trip. When I called Larry, he figured out that it was probably the Neulasta shot that I'd had after chemo to prevent my white blood cells from plummeting that had caused the spike. The doctor grudgingly accepted the explanation and handed me a prescription "just in case" of infection. He gave his reluctant blessing and wished me well.

Just before our departure, I received the news from Dr. Arnaout that my recent MRI showed no trace of cancer. The infection above my lip was starting to heal. My eyes were still watering heavily and I was low on energy, but not quite as wrecked as I had been. Even now, I can still hardly believe I got on the plane and that we arrived in Mexico, exhausted but triumphant.

There were clearly compelling reasons not to go to Mexico. It was a calculated risk that could have resulted in serious health complications. But it was worth every minute of it. It's what my mother would call "the dignity of risk," the value of making life-affirming decisions even though there may be risks and dangers. It was more important for me to go to Mexico than to cede to caution.

LETTING GO – AGAIN!

Maybe it wasn't surprising that some latent emotional issues began to surface once I got away. When I was in the thick of treatment, it felt like it was all I could do to put one foot in front of the other and get through chemo. Although there had been tears and poignant moments along the way, some of the hard stuff was no doubt lying dormant because cancer was the only front I could handle at the time.

In Oaxaca, after a few days of yakking over spectacular Mexican breakfasts with some wandering women filmmakers from Toronto, we had revealed enough about ourselves that I felt comfortable telling them I was going through breast cancer. We were able to weep together then, and later hugged as they were leaving, promising to find each other at our next stop down the coast.

A couple of days later, we traveled to Puerto Escondido. We found a restaurant near the beach for supper on our first night there, where we encountered a couple from Alberta we had met in Oaxaca who invited us to join their table. The conversation was pleasant enough, but I knew almost immediately that the talk would be light and superficial, and that this was a relationship I had little interest in pursuing. Post-diagnosis, I was becoming increasingly clear about not wanting to spend time with people simply to chitchat, as my time was too precious and possibly limited.

I imagined that Larry was feeling the same way until I heard him tell the couple that I was in the middle of breast cancer treatment. I was taken aback, hurt that he would be offering such intimate information about me to virtual strangers. Naturally, the talk then zeroed in on my cancer like a magnet, and I felt raw, exposed, and uncomfortable through the rest of the evening. I couldn't wait to get out of there.

Back at the B&B, I tearfully told l Larry how I'd felt blindsided by him at supper. He seemed surprised that I was so upset and that I'd had such a strong reaction to what had transpired, especially since I had shared my medical condition with the women in Oaxaca. Larry was confused, but I explained that I needed to be the one to decide whether to tell new people what was happening in relation to my cancer. I needed to feel safe, and if I was going to share what was going on, it would have to be with people I wanted to open up with, as I had with the women from Toronto. Cancer was my story to tell, and unless I chose to open the door first, it was off limits. It was a sensitive issue, but we had a pretty solid pact after that.

It is important for cancer patients to explain to the people we love how we feel about confidentiality and disclosure. Cancer is often new territory for everyone involved, and it's essential to put ground rules into place. The bottom line is that I needed to clearly say what would help me feel comfortable and safe, especially in social situations. I also had to communicate what wasn't working for me and what the taboos were. It was important to reach an understanding with Larry and the other significant people in my life that respected my wishes so everyone could be on the same page.

In Mexico, I was in a different place, both geographically and emotionally. For me, traveling is about more than exploring new places and cultures. It's also about traveling within and seeing myself and my relationships in new ways. Earlier, I had struggled with letting go of my work, my former identity, and my sense of myself in the world. Later, I had dealt with losing my hair and my physical well-being. In Mexico, I learned about letting go of some of my long-standing expectations.

Larry had been a closet smoker for years. When we'd met we had both smoked, but I finally quit when I was thirty and pregnant. Larry had vowed to do the same. But it didn't happen, and after that he always smoked outside, even in winter. I hated his smoking and worried about his health and our future. I'd tried not to nag Larry about it because it almost always ended in disaster, so I had learned to shut up most of the time. I tried to be strategic about how and when I pleaded with him to quit. Usually, my protests went nowhere, but occasionally he'd quit for a while. Then a few weeks or months would pass, and the telltale signs would appear that he was smoking again.

We played an unspoken game. I pretended I didn't know when Larry had started smoking again because I figured he'd smoke less if he had to hide it from me. But I'd know, and after a few months I'd finally lose it, burst into tears and beg him to quit. Once it was out in the open again, he would smoke with abandon. I began to think of Larry's cigarettes as his mistress. He'd leave the supper table or our conversations to go out and commune with her, lured by her charms.

It made me even crazier that Larry was still smoking after I was diagnosed with cancer. How could he invite cancer into his body when I was fighting so hard to get rid of it in mine? On our second night in San Augustinillo, I blew up. It had been a year since I'd said anything about his smoking, but we were living in close quarters, and I had found cigarettes in his pocket. I could no longer contain myself. It didn't make any sense to me, and I was heartbroken and furious. The dam burst. I yelled and cried. Larry became quiet and distant. I was an emotional and physical wreck afterwards.

By the next day, something had shifted. I was in a different place. It had become abundantly clear overnight that there was only one person who could quit smoking. It was an epiphany of sorts: once I let go, I became completely calm, almost serene. I didn't feel differently about the smoking, but I was at peace about what I could and couldn't do to make it happen.

I was starting to understand what the Serenity Prayer of Alcoholics Anonymous was about. Its plea to "grant me the serenity to accept the things I cannot change, the courage to change the things I can, and the wisdom to know the difference" applied not only to my relationship with Larry's smoking, but also to my relationship with cancer. Since my diagnosis, I'd tried to take charge of the things I could do something about, like putting together my team of doctors and complementary practitioners, eating well, exercising, and having good people around me.

But I also had to accept that there was a part of my cancer that would remain a mystery beyond what any science, institution, community, or family could provide. I had no influence over why I had cancer, where it might lurk in my body, or where it could go in the future. As Joyce had suggested, when I was able to accept what I could not change, influence, or fix, I could let go of fighting it. I could be at peace.

The morning after our raucous fight, the tension fizzled and Larry and I were able to find each other again. Afterwards, we were subdued as always at such moments. There was nothing more to say about the smoking. I was relieved the altercation was over and to be able to let it go. I was in a different place now that the incident, though painful, had brought a measure of calm.

For the rest of our time in Mexico, we walked the beach, explored nearby lagoons for neon-colored birds in the trees and the shadowy crocodiles lurking in the shallow water, and ate supper by candlelight under the moon. We went on a couple of hikes along the ocean into fiery sunsets. I even threw caution to the wind and swam without a bathing cap, ecstatic to feel the rush of the waves washing over my scalp.

Our sojourn in Mexico had bolstered me. I could feel my body starting to detoxify and show signs of reclaiming itself. My skin was no longer as ashen and it had picked up a bit of color. The thin layer of peach fuzz starting to sprout on my head was a sure sign that my chemo days were over. Some of my energy was starting to come back. Although my ophthalmologist had confirmed that my cataract was now ready for surgery, I could see better than I had for a while. I was grateful to finally be able to lose myself in a book.

CHAPTER SEVEN

Under the Knife: Between Hope and Despair

Once home from Mexico, it was time to get ready for surgery a week after our return. Two surgeries would take place at the same time: a lumpectomy to remove whatever remained of the lump in my left breast and a lymph node dissection in my axilla or armpit.

The prospect of breast cancer surgery felt completely different from other minor surgeries I'd had in the past. It wasn't just about fixing something gone awry in one small, contained part of me. It was about gouging out whatever remained of a virulent cancer that had infiltrated my body and might, on a whim, pick up and travel anywhere with its lethal baggage. I had horror fantasies about the surgeon's knife cutting into my breast, the flash of metal bright against my skin. The only consolation was that I wasn't facing a mastectomy.

Although procedures like mine, and even mastectomies, are generally performed as day surgeries, Dr. Arnaout said she wanted to keep me in the hospital overnight for extra support. I would have a general anesthetic that would include a pain block, a kind of epidural. I would also be on painkillers after surgery.

At the pre-op session, the nurse told me I would have a drain inserted in my underarm to get rid of the excess fluid after surgery. I would need to measure the fluid in my drain several times a day before I dumped it in the toilet. I would continue to measure it for several days until the level of fluid was less than 30 ccs over a whole day, when I would go to a clinic to have the drain removed. I was not allowed to shower as long as I had the drain.

Immediately following surgery, I was to start doing exercises to avoid lymphedema. I was to stand against a wall, extend my arm over my head, and crawl my fingers up the wall, reaching up as far as they could go. I would repeat this exercise several times a day. As I was leaving, the nurse handed me a booklet and wished me well. Though I had complete faith in my "Angel" surgeon, I dreaded what she would find deep inside me. Whatever she found would only be revealed in the pathology report that I would receive when we met three weeks later. It would tell the complete story of my cancer, how aggressive it was, and where it might take me in the future.

✉ Healing Journey #7

April 5, 2010

Dear friends and family,

There was much calamity chez nous in the days leading up to March 9th, the day of my surgery for a lumpectomy and lymph node dissection. For one thing, I saw my ophthalmologist for my recurring vision problems and learned that my previously "unripened" cataract had probably been exacerbated by chemo and now required surgery. Although I knew I would have to deal with my eye issues, the thought of another surgery on top of cancer treatment felt overwhelming.

For another thing, Larry found himself in excruciating pain on the day before my surgery, unable to urinate. As his agony continued, it became clear that he would be in no shape to be with me at the hospital. Plan B had our son Daniel and me picking up my mom and driving to the hospital, where Mom would stay with me until I went to surgery. In the meantime, Larry would work on getting an appointment with his urologist.

I was infinitely grateful to our friend Mercy, who works in the recovery room at the Queensway Carleton Hospital where my surgery was to take place. Mercy had arranged to switch to the day shift to be with me from the time I arrived at the hospital at 6:30 a.m. She had lined up her co-workers, including the admitting clerks and nurses as well as my surgeon and anaesthetist, to take special care of me. Her efforts meant that from the moment Mom and I walked through the door of the hospital, we were warmly welcomed and cared for.

After I was admitted, I was brought to the surgical prep room where I donned a gown, had my vitals checked, and got hooked up to an IV. Mercy tucked heated flannel sheets around me before she wheeled me down to a hallway outside the operating room. There, Dr. Arnaout and the anaesthetist stopped by to say hello and assure me they would do all they could to minimize my pain. In addition to the usual anaesthetic, they would be using a block that would last for a few days. I was anxious, but thankful to be in the Angel's competent hands and pleased to be her first patient of the day.

The next thing I knew, I was groggily coming to in the recovery room with Mercy standing beside me. The hours that followed are a blur of falling in and out of consciousness, sucking on ice chips, and being shown how to use a morphine pump. The nurses told me the surgery had gone well and that my room was being prepared. Hooked up to an IV and oxygen with thick bandages over my two incisions and a drain in my underarm, I was weak, dizzy, and exhausted, but relieved to know the surgery was over.

On her break, Mercy came to my room with a bouquet of red flowers, my mom arrived with yellow tulips, and Daniel strolled in with a thermos of cafe au lait. Larry told me over the phone that his urologist had catheterized him and put him on drugs to shrink his enlarged prostate. He was no longer in pain and planned to pick me up from the hospital in the morning. Thankfully, we were able to laugh and say that, between his catheter and my drain, we were "double-bagged."

It was good to be home. I was swollen and sore, but I could be up and around for the most part. I could go for short walks, do a few mild exercises to keep my arm and shoulder moving, have lunch at a vegetarian restaurant with Karen, Rachel, and my mom, and have lots of naps. I had to be careful not to put pressure on my arm getting in and out of bed, and finding a good sleeping position involved arranging pillows of various sizes in strategic places. I couldn't shower, but I managed to have baths up to my waist and to sponge bath the rest of me. Rachel even washed my nascent "hair" one day with my head hanging over the tub – I was still calling it peach fuzz, but Karen and Rachel insisted on calling it hair. The pain block plus the homeopathic remedies from my naturopath for pain and healing must have been working because I didn't need painkillers.

I keep thinking about how many times over the past eight months I've lost my body and then struggled to reclaim it. Denise says I'm like a punching bag that keeps getting knocked down and somehow rights itself again. First I lost my body to chemo, when I would feel awful for several days after each of the eight rounds, then find myself back on track for a couple of weeks before bracing for the next "hit." After my surgery, it felt like I was taking a small step toward being whole again when I had the drain removed from my underarm on Day 6. I was relieved to be less encumbered and heartened when the nurse told me I was healing well and that I must have a fabulous surgeon from the look of my incision. I could feel my energy coming back as my daily walks became longer and more confident, helped by good conversation, brilliant sunshine, and the unusually warm mid-March temperatures. I was thrilled when I could finally have my first whole body shower on Day 10. I'm sure I'll go through the yo-yo cycle again when I start radiation, knowing that it too will take its toll. But I'm grateful for my body's stubborn resilience, at least so far.

The intravenous vitamin C (IVC) treatments I receive regularly from Leesa continue to heal and sustain my body and soul. Before I started on IVC, I had passed by the room fleetingly on my way to appointments with Leesa. It's different to find myself sitting in a chair like the others now, hooked up to an IV. On my first visit, I brought the newspaper and a book on Mexico, thinking there would be lots of time to read. But I soon realized that reading would be difficult, not only because it's hard to turn the pages with an IV in your arm, but also because of what's happening in the room.

The IVC room is a tiny sunlit alcove with recliner chairs facing each other from either side of the room. There, our outstretched shoes on footrests almost touch those of the person on the other side. Four of us settle into this intimate space as Leesa plumps up our veins with hot packs, then hooks us up to our customized bags of vitamin C that hang from intravenous stands. As we will be there for the next couple of hours or so, we come armed with an assortment of water bottles, mugs of tea, snacks, reading material, cell phones, laptops, and iPods. We hope we can get through our time there without having to pee, which is possible but cumbersome with all our attachments.

Some of us are regulars, some occasional patients. We range in age from our twenties to our seventies, come from all walks of life, and are mostly women. As we are virtually all cancer patients or survivors, there is an immediate intimacy in the room besides the closeness of the space. In one way or another, we have all been to hell and back. There are no holds barred, no standing on pretence. Our stories flow like the liquid C running through our veins.

We talk about everything under the sun, like the trouble we had finding a parking spot and the vagaries of the weather. We ask each other how it's going, and hear accounts of the debilitating side effects of chemo, a discouraging MRI result, or the devastating news of a recurrence. At the same time, there are whoops of unbridled joy when one of us has a breakthrough, a good test result, or when a phase of treatment has ended. There is good-humored joking and teasing. At times we are quiet, but usually not for long. Maybe because the space is intimate and we are tethered there for almost two hours each time, we don't rush through the stories. There is time for rich detail, nuance, listening, and back and forth among this cast of ordinary/extraordinary characters who straddle the chasm between hope and despair. Here are just a few:

A beautiful theater student in her mid-twenties glows with a lust for life and wisdom beyond her years after a devastating experience with cervical cancer last year. She decided to have some of her eggs frozen in the hope of bearing a child someday, although her doctors are not optimistic because of the damage done by chemo and radiation. Her friends held fund-raising parties to help her to pay for her IVC treatments, which she now gets once a month in the hope of preventing a recurrence.

A feisty grandmother drives in from the country with her husband each week. When she had a hysterectomy last year to remove fibroids, she woke up to find that her abdomen, intestines and ovaries were riddled with ovarian cancer. Afterwards, she had chemo and radiation, made dramatic changes to her diet, and started IVC.

An accomplished lawyer discovered she had a benign brain tumor last summer. She works diligently, bringing her legal documents and sometimes her mom with her to the IVC room three times a week. As there are serious risks involved in the surgery she will need, she is trying IVC in the hope of shrinking her tumor. She loves to sing, and sometimes breaks into joyous song to the delight of all.

I don't think I realized how much angst I had been carrying around leading up to my post-op appointment with my surgeon when Dr. Angel would examine me to see how I was healing three weeks after surgery. She would also go over my pathology report and give us information on the state of my cancer. Even though my recent MRI report showed no evidence of cancer, MRI results are characterized as "just pictures" that don't necessarily tell the whole story. The pathology report, on the other hand, is based on a detailed analysis of what is going on with real tissue under a microscope, and is thus more accurate. In short, the pathology report would give me my prognosis, and I was terrified.

Larry and I arrived at the hospital with a list of questions, a notebook, and pens. We flipped aimlessly through magazines in the waiting room before Dr. Angel welcomed us into her office, apologizing for being late and for not having read my report yet as it had just come through from the pathologist. We hardly breathed, exchanging nervous glances as she pored over the document on her desk, and then watched as her face lit up with a huge smile. She told us there was no cancer found in either 1) the margins around the remnant of the cancerous tumor taken from my breast, or 2) the eighteen lymph nodes taken from my underarm (two had previously been cancerous). My prognosis was very good. The treatment had worked!

It was the best news. At the same time, it was sobering to learn that my cancer was confirmed to be a Grade 3, the highest on the aggressivity scale. When we got home, I needed quiet to absorb the information, and to sit with knowing how dire my situation had been and where my cancer could be now if I hadn't got on to the right treatment track. By the next day, I was able to revel in the good news and go to appointments with my oncologist and radiation oncologist to figure out the next steps. Their hugs and exclamations of "Fantastic!" and "It doesn't get better than this!" in response to the pathology report added icing to the cake.

I'll still need radiation. My radiation oncologist, Dr. Joanne Meng, explained that there is always the possibility of microscopic cancer cells remaining undetected in my system. If so, radiation would get them. It will also reduce my chances of a recurrence by two thirds. Radiation will start around the middle of April and I'll receive treatment five days a week for five weeks.

Sometimes described as the "least horrible" of the treatment trio of chemo, surgery, and radiation, there are still difficult side effects. Radiation can also contribute to lymphedema. But the hospital recommends an array of creams to deal with skin issues, and I'm sure Leesa will have ideas about how to get through radiation with maximum effectiveness and minimal hardship. I was pleased when I asked Dr. Meng if she would call Leesa to discuss whether I should continue to receive intravenous vitamin C during radiation, and she immediately agreed.

Larry is scheduled for surgery on April 23rd to reduce the size of his prostate. I'll have my cataract surgery on May 27th when my radiation should be over. We are hoping that by June we can celebrate the end of treatment, focus on getting strong and healthy, and enjoy summer.

Last week, Rachel proposed inviting a few of her friends for brunch while she was in Ottawa for Passover over the Easter weekend. We were delighted as they are a group of amazing young women. They are all on my Healing Journey e-mail list, so they have been traveling with me, sending lots of encouragement along the way.

As it was sunny and warm, so rare for early April, we put out the spread and arranged ourselves outside on the back deck. Rachel proposed that we "check in" with each other, a longstanding feminist practice she had learned from my mom, who had also come for brunch. Happily, Rachel too has learned that checking in is a wonderful way to bring everyone into the circle by inviting them to briefly share something of what is going on in their lives.

The check-ins were mostly about transitions: a lay-off bringing the possibility of new beginnings, going back to school, moving to a new city, finding stability after a difficult time, getting support when undergoing a medical procedure. Larry talked about his current health challenges and my mom described some of the joys and fears of old age. I told them about the good news in my pathology report and how I was starting to see the world in new ways. When I took my bandana off for them to see the new growth and said I was getting ready to face the world without a head covering, they encouraged me to step out in my minimalist coif. I think we all loved the rich exchange across three generations.

I bought shampoo today. It was an ordinary thing to do, but for me it was momentous. Even though my hair is still extremely short and takes about five seconds to dry (as opposed to the two hours it used to take), I've at least started to call it "hair." I wasn't conscious of it at the time, but it seems to me that buying the shampoo is a sign of spring, of new growth and renewal. It's something I'm not sure I would have done before getting the pathology results.

Thank you to all of you from near and far for your support in getting to this milestone in my healing journey. Your visits, e-mails, phone calls, and cards; your keen interest in what's going on; your time to walk, have lunch, or sing; your support and offers to help;

your offerings of food, rides, and knitting, your solidarity and your love have been as much a part of getting me here as any treatment. May this spring be a time of renewal for all of us.

Be well. Carpe diem.
Love, Tamara

Reflections

LOSING A PART OF OURSELVES

For centuries, excising malignant tumor(s) through surgery has been the primary intervention for those afflicted with cancer. During most of that time, surgery was the only recourse. Chemotherapy and radiation as complements to surgery only arrived on the scene in more recent decades. For breast cancer patients, surgery is generally the default. It is presumed to be the first line of attack unless there are compelling reasons to proceed otherwise. Surgery first would have been my story too, had I not landed on a better treatment path for my particular cancer.

> Dr. Shailendra Verma: "One woman, one cancer, one treatment" is still a vision. We're not there yet. In the meantime, some women will be cured by surgery while for others surgery is not appropriate. For the majority of tiny cancers, surgery is still the preferred treatment. We understand more about the cancer once we have a large amount of tissue to study in pathology, which usually means accessing the tissue through surgery. How can we study everything we need to know with the material from a tiny biopsy?

I've spoken to many breast cancer patients who, once they are diagnosed, feel a powerful need to rid their bodies of the cancer as soon as it is humanly possible. While they dread surgery and its aftermath, they believe it is more important to get the tumor(s) out before further damage or spread can take place. It is a natural and visceral response to being invaded by a potentially deadly disease.

While the rate of mastectomy has diminished in recent years, surgery still often means mastectomy for breast cancer patients. Depending on the nature of the cancer, we are sometimes offered the choice of a lumpectomy followed by radiation instead of mastectomy.

The patient may be anxious to get rid of her cancer, but losing one or both breasts is always devastating. Our breasts are intrinsically bound with our sexuality, our appearance, our identity, and our sense of self. Unlike vital internal organs like lungs or livers, they may not be biologically essential to our lives, and if we are past our childbearing years, we don't need them to feed our babies anymore. But our breasts are still wrapped up in all that we are, in our current or future relationships with our spouses or lovers, in how the world sees us and how we see ourselves.

Dr. Arnaout told me I wouldn't require a mastectomy because my tumor was located in only one part of my breast. She said that in my case, a lumpectomy and lymph node dissection followed by radiation would give me the same outcome in terms of survival as a mastectomy. I was relieved that with everything else that was happening, I'd still have some semblance of my breast at the end of it.

The other good thing about my impending surgery was that it would be less invasive because I'd gone through chemo first. A major advantage of receiving chemo before surgery was that Dr. Verma could monitor its impact on my tumors and make sure it was working. Through regular examinations of my breast and underarm, we were able to confirm that the tumors continued to shrink as I progressed through treatment. By the end of it, they appeared to have shrunk to less than half their original size, leaving far less tissue for the surgeon to remove. When it was time for surgery, the intervention would be as minimally invasive as possible. The result would be less debilitating and disfiguring.

Almost all the women in my support group had gone through mastectomies as the first step in their treatment. Some had both breasts removed, either at the same time or with a subsequent mastectomy. A few of the women told stories about unsympathetic surgeons and botched operations. One surgeon told his patient that he was going to "lop off" her breast. Often, unsightly scars, ongoing pain, and lymphedema remained. There were also stories of caring, sensitive, and highly skilled surgeons who took great care not only in excising the cancer, but also in listening to their patients and in considering their needs and how they would look and feel afterwards.

I empathized with the women who were going through mastectomies. I thought about the younger ones, the women in their thirties and forties, some with young kids. I also thought about the single women with their whole lives ahead of them, some of whom hoped to have children someday. One young woman in the group wondered aloud whether her one remaining breast would be "enough" for her husband. Others voiced fears of being shunned, rejected physically, or even abandoned by their spouses, or, if they were single, by potential new lovers yet to enter their lives. Some of the partners worked hard to support the women in their lives.

Most of the women in my support group have come to terms with having only one or no breasts, and feel that their chances of going through a recurrence have been diminished because of their mastectomies. Sometimes, they fill in one or both sides of their bras or bathing suits with prostheses on an as-needed basis, but they often feel more comfortable without them. Sometimes there is raucous humor about it when we gather: "I think that's why I'm always going to the right a little bit – I swim in circles now!" Some who chose to have a second breast removed talk about feeling liberated by their newly flattened and symmetrical chests: "You just have to go to cardio class to be glad that they're both gone!" A couple of women are considering whether to undergo surgery to have their breasts reconstructed to give them a semblance of a normal breast and achieve a yearned for symmetry following mastectomy.

RECONSTRUCTION

Reconstruction of the breast is an invasive and painful procedure. The more complex route involves taking flaps of skin from the woman's thigh, abdomen, or buttocks and using the tissue to construct a semblance of a natural-looking breast. Another route is a two-stage process that involves creating a pocket of skin in the chest wall. Several months later, a saline insert similar to the kind used in breast augmentation is implanted into the pocket. Often, a nipple and areola are tattooed onto the reconstructed breast.

A few of the women in my support group mused about whether they were willing to go through the pain and risks of reconstructive surgery. On top of everything else they were dealing with, they were weighing whether it was worth the price in pain and suffering to recreate a semblance of their former breast.

I couldn't help but wonder what it would mean to go through all of that in the hope of appearing as if nothing had changed, as if we hadn't been through the ravages of breast cancer and borne its battle scars. Who would we be doing it for? Could we pretend to "pass" as if we hadn't had the cancer? My hope was that the women who chose breast reconstruction had thought it through thoroughly and that they were doing it for themselves. I also hoped they'd wait long enough after their mastectomies to be clear about why and how they were going ahead with reconstructive surgery.

Then I met Melanie, a bright and beautiful professor in her mid-thirties who is single and loves to surf. When she was diagnosed with breast cancer, she chose a double mastectomy because of her age and family history, but she was damned if she was going to be the only woman without breasts riding her surfboard over the breakers.

Within days of her diagnosis, Melanie found out about a new procedure in which the breast cancer surgeon works in tandem with a plastic surgeon to conserve the breast skin and nipple at the time of mastectomy. Although she had to travel to a hospital in another city, Melanie has now finished many of her treatments and is pleased to be sporting two "new" breasts. She is committed, moreover, to other women having better access to a range of reconstructive choices. She is advocating that local hospitals communicate information about the options to patients and provide the necessary training and support to the surgeons to make it possible.

I believe there is no right or wrong regarding how women choose to deal with the loss of their breast(s) following mastectomy. What is important is that (1) information about the range of choices and their attendant risks and benefits be communicated to them in a clear and timely way, (2) they get the support and counseling they need to make wise and informed decisions, and (3) they make decisions based on what is best for their own physical and psychological health and well-being.

COMPLICATIONS ON THE HOME FRONT

Larry had been dealing with an enlarged prostate for a couple of years. His urologist had been monitoring him closely, and other than having to pee a lot, it seemed to be under control. He had regular PSA tests, and two biopsies had come back negative. But on the morning before the day of my surgery, Larry woke up in crisis.

I tried to talk to him and see what I could do to help, but he was so consumed with pain he could hardly speak. When a call to his family doctor yielded no more help than a suggestion to go to emergency, he shut himself in the bedroom and paced the floor like a caged animal ready to explode. It wasn't how I'd imagined the day before my surgery would be, but it was clear that Larry's priority was to see his urologist as soon as possible. In the meantime, I had to figure out how to get to the hospital for my surgery.

While Larry dealt with his own health crisis, Daniel and my mom rose to the occasion. Daniel would drive my mom and me to the hospital, and my mom would stay there with me as long as she was allowed to. Thankfully, Larry managed to arrange to see his urologist the next day.

MERCIFUL CARE

I slept fitfully that night, finally falling asleep before the alarm went off at 5 a.m. on the cold March morning of my surgery. I woke Dan up and stumbled into the shower, knowing it was my last for at least a week. As the water poured down, I looked wistfully down at the intactness of my left breast, shiny and wet as I lathered myself with antiseptic soap as instructed. I dried off quickly, got into comfortable clothes and gathered the few things I'd pulled together into an over-night bag to take with me: my rarely used cellphone, my toilet kit, a couple of button-down tops, underwear, my book. I pocketed the homeopathic remedies Leesa had recommended for pain and healing following surgery: vials of tiny pellets of arnica and hypericum to put under my tongue at regular intervals later that day. As I put my coat on, I looked around the house and wondered what shape I'd be in when I returned the next day. It felt like an eternity away.

Dan and I closed the door behind us and went out into the dark-ness to scrape the ice from the car windows. With Dan behind the wheel, we drove through the slick, empty streets to my mom's apart-ment where she was waiting for us, resolute and purposeful, ever the mother bear. We hugged briefly, then she climbed into the car and we headed across town to the hospital.

There had been several times during my cancer journey when I'd been critical of a weaknesses or incongruity within the health care system. This was especially true following my diagnosis dealing with long wait times and no treatment plan. I'd railed against the silos – each area of cancer care seemingly cut off from any others – the lack of communication and co-ordination between specialists, the cookie-cutter approach to patient care, and the absence of information and support to help newly diagnosed patients navigate the system. I'd asked a lot of tough questions. I'd written a letter to Women's Breast Health Centre at the hospital in which I recounted the details of my experience in the hope of encouraging positive change for the women who would follow me. I'd railed but I'd also tried hard to be strategic. I offered heaps of praise when it was due, raised issues, and made constructive suggestions. I hoped they'd be received in the spirit with which they were intended.

With my surgery, I had the best care I could imagine. There is no question that it was my good fortune that my friend Mercy was working as a ward assistant at the hospital. She went out of her way to take care of me and to make sure I was as comfortable as possible. But each staff person I encountered, from the admitting clerk to the nurses, the orderlies, the anesthetist, the surgeon, and the staff in the recovery room treated me with caring, respect, and skill.

At the same time, surgery is always traumatic, an attack on the body even when it's necessary and is compassionately and competently executed. When I opened my eyes in recovery, I saw a haze of uniformed bodies moving around between the beds. Attached to an IV pole with a morphine drip, I was conscious of the incisions under my bandages, one extending down from my underarm and another across my breast above the nipple. I hoped that whatever remained of my cancer had been taken out of my body, including a yet to be determined number of lymph nodes extracted from my underarm.

Although I was groggy and disoriented, it occurred to me that my tissue was probably on a cart somewhere on its way to the pathology lab. I didn't feel pain, but my left shoulder, arm, and chest were sore and uncomfortable, and I had a long thin tube coming out of my underarm that drained fluid into a clear plastic ball at the end of it. But my surgery was over. I closed my eyes and breathed a sigh of relief that the angst of anticipation was behind me as they wheeled my bed down the corridor to my room.

When Dr. Arnaout came to see me early the next morning, she asked how I had slept and how I was feeling. I told her I was surprised I wasn't in pain, that I hadn't had to use the morphine drip, and that I'd slept pretty well. I couldn't believe I was able to lift my left arm up, over and even behind my head. I said I thought I could probably even put a T-shirt on, which I'd been told I wouldn't be able to do for weeks. She said she was pleased the pain block was doing its job and explained what she had done during my surgery.

At an international conference she had recently attended, she learned a new technique called Reverse Axillary Mapping from a French surgeon who had been doing breast cancer research for years. A radioactive dye enabled her to distinguish between the lymph nodes that were exclusively draining my breast and separate them from those that exclusively drained my arm. Being able to make this distinction during my surgery allowed her to identify and preserve two of the arm lymph nodes that would otherwise have been removed unnecessarily. This operative strategy, designed to reduce lymphedema, was already doing wonders for my healing, my range of motion, and my spirits.

Dr. Angel Arnaout: The hope with this technique is to help prevent lymphedema and salvage the range of motion in the affected arm. We're going to be publishing a series of case studies of approximately twenty patients I used it with. They have all turned out fine.

I felt infinite gratitude to the Angel at that moment. But the best news was yet to come. Three weeks later, she gave us the results of the pathology report and the news that my cancer was completely gone.

STRADDLING THE BEST OF BOTH MEDICAL WORLDS

By this point, I was comfortable with how I was straddling mainstream and complementary medicine. It simply made sense: Why not take advantage of the best of what each had to offer? While chemo had been wretched, I hadn't suffered to the same extent as many women who didn't have the benefit of complementary care.

For the most part, I wasn't plagued by many of the common side effects of chemo. I'd felt queasy and weak, but I'd never vomited. The white L Glutamine powder I mixed with water, swished around in my mouth, and swallowed several times a day coated my digestive tract so that I didn't develop thrush or mouth sores. It also protected my extremities during my four rounds of Taxotere. Acupuncture before and after chemo helped me receive its benefits and counter its side effects. I was taking capsules of COQ10 (Co-enzyme Q 10) to protect my heart muscle that was battered by AC. The concentrated compounds of green tea and mushrooms I was on and the intravenous vitamin C I'd been receiving for months bolstered my immune system and aimed to fight my cancer.

Along the way, I encountered a few women with breast cancer who had decided to forego some or all of mainstream medical treatment in favor of pursuing an alternative route. One chose not to have any standard medical treatment for her cancer. Another had surgery, chemo, and radiation the first time she was diagnosed but refused to go through it again when her cancer returned. Yet another woman had surgery, but refused chemo and radiation while embracing the complementary route that included a rigorous vegan diet and exercise regimen. While I respected these choices, they had yielded mixed results. I know I wouldn't have been willing to choose one approach over the other. For me, that meant straddling, availing myself of the best each therapeutic world had to offer.

> **Dr. Leesa Kirchner:** If we were really interfering with treatment, why isn't everyone dead? Why are all these people doing so well? Why are all these cancer patients saying, "I didn't have a lot of side effects, and I'm still biking to chemo." That has to say something.

The IVC room was an oasis, a home for fellow "straddlers" like me who were looking for the best treatment possible, whatever the source.

We traded stories of our diagnoses, our doctors, our treatments, our tests, our side effects. We talked about how to get second opinions if we weren't satisfied with the first, about which doctors we liked and disliked, about approaching whatever was happening to us from

Dr. Leesa Kirchner: The people who come to me have thought this through. They rarely come to me asking, "What is it that you do exactly?"

many different angles. We met each other's families, shared recipes, books, snacks, tears, and laughter. We followed each other's progress with interest and concern. We worried if someone didn't show up for a few weeks, and were devastated if we learned that someone had lost the battle. While there were painful moments, it felt good to be among such kindred spirits, each of us searching, asking questions, unwilling to leave any stone unturned in our quest to heal and be well.

CHAPTER EIGHT

Radiation:
Close to the Finish Line, and Yet...

It was April and spring was in the air, bringing signs of new life as the bleakness of the long winter months melted away. It felt like things were starting to look up. There was a spring in my step as I discovered anew the joys of the daytime world. Chemo and surgery were behind me. The results of my pathology report were hopeful. My scars were healing, looking less angry and red. Everyone who saw them, particularly those with some level of expertise or experience, commented on the stellar job my Angel surgeon had done. So far, I had no signs of lymphedema. There was evidence that my trusty hair follicles were readying themselves to make a comeback in their own capricious, unpredictable way. I turned fifty-nine, not particularly a landmark birthday, but for me it was momentous. I was here. I was doing all right, with significantly more reason to hope than a few months before. I was more determined than ever to embrace my life for whatever amount of time I had left.

After the rollercoaster ride of the previous eight months, the thought of going through radiation felt relatively benign. Primarily preventive, I imagined it would be the least invasive and the most tolerable of the treatments I'd have to endure. It would also be the last of the troika. It would be time-consuming but manageable to get to the hospital for radiation. Debbie and Denise were already busy lining up a schedule for my team of drivers.

I was pleased when Dr. Meng, my radiation oncologist, readily agreed to call Leesa to discuss whether I should continue to receive intravenous vitamin C during radiation. After their conversation and reading the literature, Dr. Meng wasn't convinced that the IVC wouldn't act as an antioxidant and thus interfere with the benefits of radiation, but she left the decision to me. I stewed about it for a few days before finally deciding to suspend IVC during radiation.

When Dr. Meng told me that excessive fatigue and burning and blistering of the skin were common side effects of radiation, I was able to take her ominous warning and tuck it away for future reference. I was thrilled when she said I could keep on swimming as long as my skin was holding up. I took a deep breath. Five weeks from now, my marathon of treatment would be behind me and I could start working on getting strong and healthy again.

Once I was set up with my markers, the small tattoos that would position me for each treatment, I started my radiation routine. Every day, one of my dedicated Rad Rider friends would arrive to take me to treatment. We would drive the twenty minutes or so to the hospital, park the car, walk through the doors of the center and head down the hallway. I'd greet the staff at the desk and swipe my card to let the system know I'd arrived. Then I'd go into a small cubicle to change into a blue cotton hospital gown. I'd come back to the waiting room to sit and chat with my driver, and then one of the two young technicians who would be working with me would call me in.

Arriving in the cavernous radiation chamber, they'd check my birth date to make sure they had the right person. I'd undo the ties on my gown to expose my breast, looking down on it as I made a silent wish for it to receive the radiation as healing rays. I'd climb up on to the platform and lie down on my back with my left arm above my head, closing my eyes while I tried to be as still as humanly possible while the technicians set up the equipment. When the machines were precisely programmed and positioned, the technicians would leave the chamber, and I'd be alone while gigantic electronic eyes beamed their rays down on me. I'd try to zone out, usually without much luck, wishing I'd taken meditation more seriously. After about ten minutes, the technicians would return and help me down from the platform. I'd slip my gown back on, and head back to the cubicle to slather my breast, underarm, shoulder, and neck with the creams Leesa had recommended.

Once a week after my treatment, Larry and I would sit in the waiting area until a nurse ushered us into an examining room. Then Dr. Meng would arrive in her white lab coat, clutching my file close to her chest. She'd be hurried and sometimes breathless, but always beaming with a smile that lit up her face. She would ask how I was doing and whether I had any chest pain or shortness of breath before closely examining the areas of my body that had been radiated. Other than a bit of redness that developed after the first few weeks of treatment, my skin seemed to be holding up. Dr. Meng's warning about excessive fatigue hadn't yet materialized.

✉ Healing Journey #8

July 6, 2010

Dear friends and family,

In early April, I shed my headgear for good, spurred on by the encouragement of Rachel and her friends when we spent time together over the Easter/Passover weekend. At last, I was ready to go out into the world unencumbered by wigs, bandanas, scarves, and hats. It was time. Of course, I didn't have my mane of thick, long hair, but it felt okay to have a close crop of soft gray "puppy" hair for now. I even got compliments on my new "hairstyle," and was surprised to hear from the kids that some young women in their twenties are actually choosing to dye their hair gray! My first swim in the Y pool without a bathing cap for camouflage felt almost orgasmic.

A month after surgery, Larry and I met with my radiation oncologist, Dr. Joanne Meng, who explained the benefits of radiation. She also took time to answer our questions, to tell us that skin burning and fatigue were likely side effects of radiation, especially toward the end of treatment, and that they were cumulative. There could also be other complications in rare cases. My radiation treatments would start on April 16th.

We decided to make a weekend trip to New York to see Larry's family before the start of radiation and Larry's prostate surgery. I was pleased to discover that even though it had been a while since I'd seen the family, some of them had been reading my Healing Journey letters throughout. It felt like they were there with me, almost as if we had been through the experience together with a new level of intimacy that had grown over time. I know it wouldn't have been the same if I'd tried to recount my stories in the present. My sister-in-law Nisa, who went through her own struggle with breast cancer a dozen years ago, shared a quote from Albert Camus: "In the midst of winter,

I finally learned that there was in me an invincible summer." I'm trying to hold on to that one.

My friends Debbie and Denise generously offered to step up to the plate again, inviting the Supper Sisters, with some new additions, to prepare and deliver meals to us twice a week. They also organized a dedicated team of "Rad Riders" to pick me up and drive me to the hospital five days a week for five weeks. This outpouring of generosity meant that there would be both invaluable practical support and a chance for short but delicious visits.

Before radiation, I had my "markers" done at the hospital. This involved lying on a platform while, under the direction of Dr. Meng, technicians determined the precise position I would need to be in to receive the positive impact of radiation with the least amount of damage. The tiny tattoos marking the areas of my body to be targeted were then incorporated into my personal radiation plan prepared by Dr. Meng.

As I approached the first session, I couldn't help but notice how ill some of the patients in and around the waiting room seemed to be. Often, they were in hospital beds or wheelchairs. I found myself being grateful for how well I was feeling and for my level of energy.

The first session was somewhat daunting, although the technicians did their best to be warm and welcoming. I was ushered into a large, space-age room with huge pieces of equipment looming from the ceiling and asked to lie on a hard platform in the middle of the room. Two technicians then worked to position me precisely with my left arm raised above my head as they called out measurements to each other and entered them into a computer. Then they left for the control room to operate the machines that would radiate me. My main challenge was to lie as still as possible and try to resist any urge to sneeze or scratch before the treatment ended.

After a few days, the sessions became almost routine. The daily visits with my Rad Riders were special moments in my days and I continued to feel good, walking, swimming, working out at the Y, seeing friends. I slathered on skin cream several times a day to protect the areas of my body that were being radiated. Larry had his prostate surgery, and was relieved to come home the next day without a catheter and able to urinate on his own for the first time in almost two months. That night, unencumbered at last, we booked tickets to Greece for September, the dream trip I'd wistfully hoped could be my prize at the end of treatment.

I turned fifty-nine on April 22nd, a birthday like no other. I was here. It was a birthday I didn't know I'd have, or for which I could have been very sick had my treatment not got on the right track at the eleventh hour. It was also my first birthday without my dad. It was sobering that he was gone now, but I was grateful to be feeling well and able to celebrate in a low-key way.

Dr. Meng was pleased with how I was doing and how my skin was holding up when I saw her at our weekly appointments. On one visit after she had examined me, she asked what I'd be doing for the rest of the day. When I told her I'd be getting together with a couple of friends that afternoon to sing, she was intrigued, and wanted to know more about what I was doing to get through treatment. I told her about Missy singing me through chemo and about my Healing Journey letters. I told her how the writing was therapeutic for me and how my friends and family felt more included in the experience because of it. I promised to send her a copy. I also told her how the Supper Sisters and the Rad Riders were part of my amazing community in Ottawa and beyond that were supporting me in so many ways.

I was worried about my eyesight. My vision was getting worse because of the advanced state of a cataract on my good eye that had been exacerbated by Taxotere. Reading, writing, and e-mailing were becoming increasingly strained, which I found especially hard as a book lover, would-be writer, and long-time literacy worker. Driving was starting to involve too much guesswork. With cataract surgery scheduled for May 27th, I decided it was no longer safe to drive.

But I was so close to the finish line I could taste it. My pathology report had shown I was cancer free, and I was feeling good at almost the end of four of my five weeks of radiation and the end of treatment. Soon I'd be able to see well, read, and drive again. I was looking forward to summer and to getting strong and healthy again.

The day after I stopped driving was sunny and warm, the lilacs in full bloom. Debbie and I were meeting Judy for her birthday breakfast on Elgin St. and I had a meeting at Inter Pares afterwards, so I decided my bike would be the best way to get around town. The ride along the canal was glorious, the scent of lilacs everywhere. Laughing and crying as we commiserated over the disappointments of our respective Mother's Days, we toasted the freedoms of being "of a certain age." I rode on to Inter Pares, appreciating how non-plussed staffers were when I asked them to read the agenda out loud to me in my non-literate state. At the end of our meeting, I noticed that my chest was feeling tight, but didn't think much of it. But as I rode home, my breathing became increasingly labored as the pain closed in around my chest like a vice grip. As soon as I got home gasping and barely able to breathe, we headed for the emergency room.

As a radiation patient, there was no wait time. Emergency staff administered a series of tests that ruled out the more dreaded possibilities: a heart attack, blood clot, return of my cancer. They figured that what happened was probably caused by the radiation, as the radiated area of my body included my heart and lungs as unwitting targets even though every effort had been made to protect them. Once my breathing was restored, Dr. Meng recommended continuing radiation as long as I had no further chest pain. But a couple of days later, the chest pain was back and we ended radiation for good. I'd received twenty-two out of the twenty-five treatments that had been planned.

I wish I could say I went dancing in the streets to celebrate the end of treatment. I was pleased to be done with it, of course, but it all felt tentative for some reason. I wasn't quite ready to dance yet.

Victoria Day was approaching, and we headed to the cottage for the weekend where Rachel and Daniel would join us. But each day I was there I got weaker, and found myself spending more and more time collapsed in bed. On Monday, after nearly passing out in the shower, we headed back to emergency.

I was so weak, apparently, because my heart was racing at double its normal rate. The doctors brought my heart rate down with the drug Adenosine, put me on oxygen, and monitored me around the clock. An echocardiogram and chest X-ray showed excess fluid around my heart and lungs that was getting in the way of my breathing and heart function, a fairly unusual complication from radiation. After four days, I was sent home with beta blockers to keep my heart rate down.

My time at home, however, was short-lived. Karen was visiting from Toronto, and it felt good just to sit in the backyard relaxing and playing Upwords. But when I woke up from a nap in the early evening chilled and sweating with a 104-degree fever, we headed back to emergency again.

This time, a slew of doctors tried to figure out what was going on and what kind of infection had caused my fever. Oncologists, cardiologists, respirologists, and infectious disease specialists examined me and ran all kinds of tests. Blood cultures produced inconclusive or negative results. They considered draining the fluid from my lungs, but decided against it, hoping my body would get rid of it naturally. Dr. Meng visited me often, caring and attentive but as baffled as her colleagues. I was terrified that the cancer had returned when excruciating pain developed in my left hip, but that possibility was ruled out by an X-ray. A strange rash began to develop on my left calf before I was discharged after spending a total of ten days in hospital.

Four days after leaving hospital, my family doctor diagnosed shingles, the dormant chicken pox virus that strikes when the immune system is compromised. After going through chemo and radiation, I was an easy target. I hated having to cancel so many of the things I had hoped to do in June, but I had to accept that I was incredibly weak, that I had lost fifteen pounds in two weeks, and that I was suffering from shingles. I had canceled the appointment for cataract surgery when I was in hospital, so my vision was still a problem. I had to miss the June Inter Pares board meeting and the New Arts Festival where Larry was selling his woodturnings. I couldn't be at the Spirit of Rasputin's tribute evening of Songs of Protest, Songs of Hope in honor of my dad, or at Louise's retirement party. I'd have to miss the annual tradition of going to the Shaw Festival in Niagara-on-the-Lake with my mom and Karen, and we postponed Kathryn and Al's visit to the cottage from Vancouver Island.

It was hard not to be discouraged as my world became increasingly small, compounded by not being able to read or drive myself to appointments. All through treatment, my body had worked hard to stay resilient and strong. There could be several rotten days, but then somehow it would rally and bounce back. This time, it was as if my body had screamed "Enough!" with the cancer and the treatments. I felt a new kinship with the infirm cancer patients I had seen in the waiting room.

For the first time, it was a challenge to think about walking a couple of blocks or climbing a staircase. I had to learn to be (a) patient. Dr. Meng called several times a week to see how I was doing. The shingles pain was constant, which meant I didn't sleep well at night and that I needed to nap at least twice a day. I had such low stamina that I couldn't plan visits unless they were tentative, spaced wide apart, and short. My mom was my devoted and constant visitor during this time. I tried to listen to books on tape and Larry and I played a lot of Upwords, with Larry having to look up words that I couldn't read in the dictionary.

In spite of everything, there were special moments. There was time with friends in Ottawa as well as from out of town who had been supportive from a distance. My Brujas ("Witches" in Spanish) sisters had planned to visit from Toronto and Winnipeg when I thought I'd be well on the road to recovery by mid-June. Although I badly wanted to see them, I was weak and depleted and didn't know if I could handle it. It was only when they said "We want to come even if it's only for half an hour" that I felt able to confirm, and we had brief but glorious visits one late afternoon and the next morning.

Our daughter Rachel has been a constant source of love and support through this "year from hell," as we have come to call it. An avid cyclist living in Montreal, she and her friends created a bike-a-thon "Ride Beside/Côte-à-Côte" to cycle from Montreal to Ottawa to raise money for Wellspring, which provides non-medical support for people with cancer and their families.

Seven riders and their support crew arrived at our house, tired but exhilarated the afternoon of June 26th. After showers and time to relax, we had supper brought in and toasted the Ride Besiders before they partied and crashed on beds, couches, and camping mats all over our house. I slept at my mom's that night, thrilled but completely exhausted. Thanks to so many of you and others, they surpassed their goal of $10,000.

My shingles are on the wane and recent tests show that the fluid around my heart is gone, which means the fluid around my lungs should be gone too. By the droplet, I seem to be getting a bit stronger each day. I was able to get a new appointment for cataract surgery for July 7th, and while I'm not looking forward to the surgery, I can't wait to see well again. We are all looking forward to the "year from hell" being over, aiming for July 31st and getting to the Blue Skies Folk Festival, exactly a year after my diagnosis.

I want to thank so many of you near and far for your cards, letters, and messages and for your constant support and generosity expressed in so many ways during this time.

May you have a wonderful summer.

Be well. Carpe diem.
Love, Tamara

Reflections

CIRCLES OF SUPPORT

When radiation treatment began, I knew I could have driven myself to the hospital. But I appreciated spending time with my driver friends who offered me daily doses of support and companionship. As my eyesight gradually worsened, I realized it was no longer safe for me to drive and that their help was now a requirement. Thankfully, the Rad Riders were lined up and raring to go.

It was a big deal for me to learn how to ask for and receive help. I was the classic elder child, the responsible one, better at giving and caretaking than at receiving support. But with cancer, I learned the hard way that the absurd notion of being strong and self-sufficient is a sorry and misguided illusion none of us can sustain. There was no more being "strong," only the raw, naked truth of what was happening to me. I came to see my vulnerability as a surprising but precious source of strength. The more deeply I was able to recognize, accept, and share some of my vulnerabilities with others, the more I could see that they too were relieved to be able to open up in new ways about their own foibles and anxieties. In the process, we would inevitably reach a new level of intimacy and friendship, all pretense gone by the wayside. Somewhere along the way, I started to feel more worthy of being loved and cared for.

Being able to receive with an open heart was part of acknowledging and even embracing my vulnerability. But it was something I had to learn how to do. I had a choice. I could accept the offers of help, support, and friendship flowing my way, or I could discourage them and deal with cancer on my own or only with those closest to me. Once I decided it was better to receive, albeit selectively, it got easier with practice. As I got better at it, I realized that receiving is like vulnerability. Giving/receiving and strength/vulnerability are essentially flip sides of the same coins. With practice, each side merges into and becomes the other, and both aspects of our selves are the better for it.

SOME PRACTICAL MATTERS ABOUT SUPPORT SYSTEMS

When cancer strikes, it affects everyone in our world at the same time. The news of our illness means the dreaded sword they all fear has fallen once again upon yet another friend, colleague, neighbor, or family member. Everyone is terrified but also threatened when they hear the news. While they understand that cancer is happening to us, they also see it as happening to them. The spin of the roulette wheel has spared them, *but only this time.*

They express their fear in different ways: with avoidance, discomfort, awkwardness, anguish, love, empathy, and compassion, or some combination thereof. Often, they badly want to be able to do something, anything to help fix things or at least make life a bit easier or more comfortable. If they are ready and willing to be there to help in meaningful ways, it can be a win-win result for all concerned.

As patients, we need as much practical support as we can get. We may be surprised to see that the people in our lives are grateful to be doing something useful and to feel needed and appreciated for their efforts. But we don't necessarily welcome help with open arms. There is a fine line between what kind of support is wanted or will be welcomed and what is not wanted or appropriate. Those around us must respect that the patient has to call the shots about whether, who, what, how, and when help is needed. Sometimes, it is a question of timing. Support that might not be needed or wanted at one point may be welcomed and appreciated later on. The support can take many forms. It can involve helping out with:

- preparing food, delivering meals, grocery shopping

- driving/accompanying the patient to medical and other appointments

- arranging or providing childcare

- arranging for or doing housecleaning, yard work, and other chores

- running errands or making phone calls

- doing research

- giving, lending, or raising money

- brainstorming, troubleshooting, and problem solving with the patient and her family

- being available to hang out, sit together in silence, or go for a walk.

It helps when a friend volunteers to co-ordinate the team. Two organizers are even better, if possible. Sometimes friends, neighbors, and colleagues generously offer their services and wait to be called upon, but this generosity can wane if it isn't soon harnessed. The patient needs to feel comfortable with whomever is playing the role of co-ordinator(s) to organize a variety of tasks, such as:

- discussing possibilities for help with the patient and figuring out what she wants and needs

- assembling e-mail addresses and writing e-mail messages and responses

- organizing schedules and putting the completed calendar together

- being the contact person if changes need to be made

- thanking the team.

The conversations I had with my Rad Riders were often the social highlight of my day. Although I was independent in many ways, it made a huge difference to know I wasn't alone. Some of the patients who populated the waiting room had another person there with them; others were alone. I was always grateful to have someone by my side.

My friends told me how pleased and relieved they were to be able to do something concrete. It worked both ways. It meant the world to me to have a meal waiting at the end of the day and a friend in the waiting room, to yak about what was going on with each of us, or just to sit together in silence.

CUMULATIVE COMPLICATIONS

I was well into my fourth week of radiation when I decided it was finally time to stop driving. I probably should have stopped sooner because of my diminishing vision, but I'd been reluctant to give up the freedom of having my own wheels. It was almost the middle of May, only ten days away from the end of treatment, and other than the problems with my eyesight, I was feeling good. If successful, my cataract surgery would get to the root of my vision problems and restore my vision. Meanwhile, I had a busy morning and I wanted to try out my bike.

It was a bitter irony that my first day on my bike started out so well and ended so badly. It was gloriously liberating to ride along the canal to the restaurant on Elgin Street. With several activities planned, I was ready to don my helmet and ride from one encounter to the next. A couple of hours later after a harrowing ride home, I let my bike drop with a crash in the backyard before I stumbled into the house, doubled over and hardly able to breathe. I was seized with a double terror. Was the cancer spreading to my lungs? If not, what was going on?

Thankfully, Larry was home and could take me to emergency. As soon as the nurses found out I was a radiation patient, they whisked me into a bed, put me on oxygen, and started tests.

It seemed that what had befallen me was an unfortunate convergence of the cumulative effects of radiation and the impact of a new physical activity. The emergency staff gave me oxygen and drugs for my breathing and chest pain over the next several hours before they sent me home. I had six radiation sessions left.

When the chest pains returned, Dr. Meng agreed I'd had enough with 90 percent of the benefits radiation could offer me. When I asked her whether she had seen reactions like mine before, she said she had, but it was rare. The powerful beams were targeting my left breast, putting my heart and left lung in the line of fire. They had become inflamed in response to radiation as my heart labored to keep pumping blood and my left lung to keep breathing. With each organ working twice as hard to do its job, the result was shortness of breath, weakness, and chest pain.

A few days after stopping radiation, I was so weak I could hardly walk. When we went back to emergency, we learned that my heart rate had gone

> Dr. Joanne Meng: Your body was injured in response to the radiation. It's very rare. I can think of only one other person who had the same thing and was treated with anti-inflammatories. When the inflammation settled, your body was able to fight the inflammation and the fluid was reabsorbed.

through the roof, pumping at more than double its normal speed. Now that I had a more serious case of pericarditis and pulmonary edema, excess fluid on my heart and lung, they hooked me up to a labyrinth of tubes and machines to try to bring my heart rate down. Nurses and doctors constantly came in and out of my urgent care cubicle, monitoring me around the clock.

After midnight, I was dozing, when a team of nurses descended. A monitor showed that my heart rate was spiking again, and they were there to give me an emergency injection and set me up on an intravenous drip to bring it down. Drugged and dopey, it felt like a frenzied SWAT team had swooped down on me. A nurse grabbed my left arm and I protested, begging her to use my portocath or my right arm instead for the IV. I told her I was in danger of developing lymphedema if I received injections or IV, had blood taken, or had my blood pressure checked on that side because of the lymph node dissection in my left underarm. The nurse replied curtly that this was an emergency, and they would do whatever they had to do to deal with the situation. I closed my eyes, gritting my teeth as she proceeded to push the IV into a vein in my left arm. I wept silently after the nurses left the room, feeling weak and helpless. I tried to sleep, but I felt like a giant octopus with all the tubes dangling in and out of me, and it was hard to get comfortable with the lights on.

The next day, I was admitted to the cardiology unit. I'd always had a strong heart, but I'd been through four rounds of the combined chemo drug AC, which is especially hard on the heart. Now, my heart was fighting the battle of its life after being repeatedly assaulted by chemo and radiation.

Dr. Meng came to see me whenever she could. She seemed flustered and worried, mystified about what was happening to me. I know she did everything in her power to make sure I got good care. After four days, I was discharged and sent home, armed with beta-blockers to keep my heart rate down. But eight hours later I was back in emergency, shivering and weak with a high fever, hooked up to the tubes and machines again. This time, they were trying to figure out what was causing the fever.

The doctors never solved the mystery of what caused my fever during the week I spent in hospital. Maybe there were just too many things wrong with me at the same time. While all my symptoms appeared at various points over the course of my stay, it was my family doctor who made the diagnosis just a few days after discharge: I had shingles.

It is the nature of the shingles virus for its symptoms, if they are multiple, to appear sequentially. In my case, it started with the fever followed by almost unbearable pain in my hip a few days later, and then the rash on my calf. Often, a rash is the only visible symptom, usually accompanied by nerve pain. Apparently, it's only when the constellation of earlier possible symptoms combines with the rash that a diagnosis of shingles can be made.

I was an easy target for shingles, the virus that had been lurking in my nerves for decades after an early bout of chicken pox. I returned home and retreated into my ever-shrinking, semi-literate, and cloistered world of nerve pain, infirmity, and visual impairment.

What can you do when you are caught in a cascade of relentless attacks on the body and spirit? Some people turn to faith at this point and seek comfort in their beliefs. While this wasn't my inclination, I found myself thinking about what I knew of Job, a good man who suffered terribly, losing his children and possessions and enduring immense pain and suffering including boils (shingles?) over a long period of time. Job is renowned for his patience and faith in the face of great adversity.

While I didn't seek out religion, I thought about what I'd learned from Joyce early on in the cancer experience. This was the mantra I practiced: "I'm getting the best possible care available from the health care system. I'm doing everything possible that naturopathic oncology has to offer me. I'm eating as well as I can (in spite of the tasteless hospital food) and trying to take care of myself. My family and friends are here for me. People far and wide are praying, chanting, meditating, singing, and sending me their positive energy. In short, I'm doing all that I can to heal and be well. I have to accept that the rest is a mystery."

This way of understanding spirituality resonated for me, but there were still moments of doubt when I thought about giving up the fight. Then I'd lie in the hospital bed with my eyes closed to keep out the glaring lights, and think about what I'd been through and all I had to live for. Somehow, I'd find a few new ounces of strength to carry on, at least for that moment.

THE COUNTRY OF OLD AGE

When I was in hospital the second time, I shared a room with an elderly woman who was asleep most of the time. Her head was small and feathery, almost bird-like, and she was breathing heavily. Nurses came to her bedside, made adjustments to her IV and left quietly, but she kept on sleeping. The only thing I knew about her was that her name was Irene.

A young man arrived to visit with her. He pulled up a chair to sit close beside her, leaning over and speaking to her with warmth and affection, as engaged as if she were alert and responsive. He hooked up an iPod that played beautiful classical music, and spoke to her animatedly about composers and symphonies. Later, he came over to talk to me.

Irene was his grandmother. She was ninety-nine years old. She had been living in a retirement residence, doing pretty well until she became dehydrated and was taken to hospital. The young man was one of her four grandsons, the children of Irene's only daughter who had died when the boys were young. He had come from Toronto to see her, and told me Irene was a concert pianist and piano teacher who was like a mother to them. She had clearly passed on her love of music to the boys.

His brothers came to visit Irene too. One grandson asked if she knew what would happen when she turned one hundred. "Guess what, Grandma," he said. "You're going to get a letter from the queen!" Another teased her, quizzing her about which of Rachmaninoff's concertos was playing on the iPod. Over the next few days, Irene seemed to rally a bit. She was more alert and able to sit up in her chair for short periods, drink sips of a meal supplement, and visit with her grandsons.

Looking across to Irene's side of the room, it occurred to me that I was encroaching on her territory. Here I was, a full forty years her junior, but I felt like I was dipping my toe into her country. I was weak after all that had happened, my energy depleted, and my strength at an all-time low. It was frustrating to have to cancel the cataract surgery, and I didn't know when it could be rescheduled. Once I was unplugged from my various tubes, I was usually able to read the computer screen and do some e-mailing, but I could still barely read a book or newspaper. I wondered what had become of my old "piss and vinegar," that had always bounced back to sustain me, even in my darkest hours. Would it ever return?

Although we hardly talked, I felt Irene and I had some important things in common. I figured that each of us, in our own way, was reckoning with our respective frailties and our precarious relationship with the Grim Reaper. Late one night when the ward had quieted down, I sat next to her bed and sang "Goodnight Irene" as she slept peacefully. Two months after I left the hospital, I read Irene's obituary in the newspaper. She hadn't quite made it to one hundred to get her letter from the queen, but I hoped she'd had a "good death."

I talked to my mother about Irene, and how I thought I had been living in the country of old age during the last few weeks. I asked her if it was the same territory she had spent the last while learning to inhabit. My trip there, which started with the complications from radiation, was marked by many of the realities that visit the old: constant pain, endless waiting, loss of freedom, no control, fear of the unknown, the need to grudgingly learn to be (a) patient. Like the old, I came face to face with my mortality.

Visiting old age was different from the angst of learning I had an aggressive cancer. Then, although I was in shock, my body felt strong and resilient, "normal." Now, there was such unfamiliar physical weakness, infirmity, and pain that I wondered if I was losing my life force. Is "life force" the physical manifestation of one's will to live?

When I lost my energy, my appetite (hunger?), my desires, I asked myself, *Is this what it means to be old? Is this what dying feels like?*

The weakness, so different from tiredness or fatigue, was a state I had previously only glimpsed when I was sick with the flu, when I'd wonder if I had the strength to get up from bed to go to the bathroom. Then, knowing I'd feel better in a few days, I'd think, *This is what it will be like when I'm old.* But now, the weakness and pain lingered on, stripped my muscles of their strength as they slackened, took my vision, left me vulnerable to the ravages of shingles, robbed me of sleep, and flattened me in ways I had never known before.

CHAPTER NINE

Healing:
Turning a New Leaf

I was both excited and terrified to finally be going ahead with the cataract surgery, rescheduled for early July. I was terrified at the thought of having such a delicate operation, although from most accounts, I'd heard it was pretty much a straightforward procedure with few complications. But I'd also spoken to others who'd had various difficulties. Although I knew the risks were minimal, I worried. I had little choice. If I had any hope of seeing well again, I'd have to go through with it.

Being able to see again felt like it could be the start of new beginnings in my life. I hadn't expected it would happen so soon after the operation. It was as if a thick layer of fog had been wiped off my eyes, opening up a new world of color, texture, and detail in everything around me. Although I had to put drops in my eyes several times a day and avoid lifting and swimming for a while, I was over the moon. It struck me that my vision was not only better than it had been before going through chemo, it was better than it had been in many years.

Being able to see again also felt like spring revisited. Could this mean that I was turning a corner, that my "year from hell" might be coming to an end? Was my body finding a source of strength to rally in new ways, choosing vitality over sickness and infirmity? Was there hope that I could recover and get some semblance of my life back? Did I want my old life back or were there things about it I wanted to change? Could "re-covery" also be about "re-invention?"

When my mom and I decided to pick up our correspondence, she wrote: "You sound so light and upbeat…. How wonderful it feels to hear that tone, to sense that mood. It's not that I don't want to hear the tough side of life – I want to hear all sides of you, the bitter and the sweet, the interesting and the boring, the joys and the sorrows. Just to let you know, dear, that I am revelling in your wellness, whenever it's there."

Her words, as always, were thoughtful and wise. It was true that life is both bitter and sweet at the same time. Having gone through the ordeal of the last year, I knew that every moment of my life was becoming infinitely more sweet and precious. I was in love with life again.

✉ Healing Journey #9

August 16, 2010

Dear friends and family,

I had my cataract surgery on July 7th. Although I could barely stomach the thought of yet another medical intervention, I couldn't wait to be able to see well again. But I worried, because even though most people have positive experiences with cataract surgery, there are still risks. What if there were complications? What if it didn't work?

Thankfully, my fears dissolved soon after I received my new lens. I was thrilled on the drive home from the hospital to be able to read the license plate on the car in front of us. I could see the bright red and green of the traffic lights, which I'd been barely able to distinguish before. I could pick up the newspaper and read beyond the headlines, and think about which book I would choose to read from my tottering pile that had been growing over the past non-reading months. The flowers in the back garden appeared startlingly vivid and beautiful, as if I was seeing them this way for the first time. On the other hand, I found wrinkles and sags in my face I didn't know I had! I could drive for the first time in almost two months. I felt like my world had gone from one of fuzzily muted pastels to brilliant technicolor, and I could see even better than before. I was immensely grateful to have had the surgery, and wondered what my fate would have been had I lived in a third world country, where I might slowly have gone blind.

But the joy of seeing well again was tempered by the constant leg pain that continued to plague me. I had fallen trying to navigate my way down a steep hill at the cottage on the Canada Day weekend and messed up my left knee, the same leg that was weak and still wracked by the lingering nerve pain of shingles. I was limping badly, finding walking and especially climbing stairs difficult, and needed to borrow a cane from my mom. I slept fitfully, waking several times during the night, unable to fall back to sleep for hours at a time because of the relentless pain. My sleep deprivation was getting in the way of healing that was taking far too long, and I felt a kinship with those who live with chronic pain. I wondered whether my body was capable of healing itself yet again after all it had been through.

In mid-July, I was glad to make it to my breast cancer support group, especially since I'd missed the previous encounter when I was too weak to get there. It was a new foray for me, as I had been mostly reclusive since the complications from radiation had begun two months before. I'd often been too weak for visits unless they were short and spaced out, hardly venturing into the outside world.

As we'd long since finished our six-week program at the hospital last fall, we were now getting together for our monthly lunch in a round (essential!) booth at a restaurant, where we check in to see where everyone is at. It's been an important group of women for me, even though my "bosom buddies" are not part of the rest of my life. The truth is that we have shared such a life-altering experience that in some ways, we understand what each other has been through better than anyone else.

Coming from diverse backgrounds and stages of life and ranging from our mid-thirties to our mid-seventies, we've shared tips on finding doctors who are both competent and human (and avoiding those who aren't) and strategies for getting through treatment. It's been a place where we can vent and share what's really going on, like when one woman told us how losing her hair was harder than losing her breast and another wondered how to tell her young children about her cancer. When I e-mailed the group in May to let them know I had landed in hospital, I got a slew of heartfelt messages back.

At lunch, a couple of the women were starting to think about going back to work. Still weak and needing at least one nap a day, I tried to imagine what it would be like to return to work. For me, the thought of working even one day a week feels daunting, and it is clear I still have a long way to go to get strong and healthy again.

After my cataract surgery, we started spending more time at the cottage. On a quiet canoe lake in Val des Monts, Quebec, an hour outside Ottawa, it is a sanctuary where the separation between being there and "in the world" is always palpable.

This summer, the cottage has been my place to heal, especially once I could read again, and I spend my days reading, staring at the lake, napping, playing Upwords. The quiet of the woods, punctuated by the haunting call of the loon, is soothing, and the lake water is velvety smooth, smelling of rocks and trees. I was determined to build up my strength by swimming each day, and as I took my first tentative strokes, the water felt encouragingly buoyant, almost amniotic, holding and propelling me as if willing me to swim farther and stronger. Once I stopped limping, I started to walk my familiar route down the dirt road, picking wildflowers. I made small gains each day toward my goal of reaching (and hitting) the stop sign at the end of it, my 5K meditative constitutional of so many years.

I'd leave the cottage for a couple of days each week to go to medical appointments, to see my mom, and as my energy began to increase, to see some of the friends who feed my soul. It's good, after the long hiatus, to be able to get together with a friend, to sit in the garden and catch up over coffee, go for a walk, or even meet for lunch. I still make virtually no evening plans, however, as I know my strength will have long waned by then. After my stint in the city, I head back to the cottage as I cross over into my other world of calm and natural wonder.

We had planned to go to the Blue Skies folk festival on the August long weekend. For the last twenty years, we had built our summer plans around Blue Skies, hungry to return for the music and the community spirit there. We would be camping for four days this time and had committed to volunteer in the kitchen, where we would help prepare meals during the festival. It would also be the anniversary of getting the news of my cancer diagnosis, and it seemed fitting to mark it at Blue Skies.

But as the time for Blue Skies grew nearer, I wondered whether to go. My energy had only just begun to return and my stamina was limited, especially as the day wore on. I worried that I wouldn't have it in me to help do the shopping, cooking, packing, shlepping, and set up involved in camping, or to make the trek to the outhouse each night especially if the weather was hot or wet. I probably wouldn't last through the evening concerts let alone be able to do the rounds of musical campfires late into the night. As much as I wanted to be there, it became clear that it wasn't worth risking a setback. I was disappointed to miss Blue Skies, but I was at peace with our decision.

As I write this, I feel my life force starting to return. Last week, the cardiologist said I had responded well to treatment. The fluid around my heart is gone, my heart is healthy, and I'm off the beta-blockers I'd been on since hospital. This means I am now on no drugs. My energy is slowly coming back, along with my appetite, stamina, and my will to get strong and healthy.

At the cottage on July 31st, the anniversary of the fateful day of my diagnosis, Larry, my mom, Daniel, and I toasted the end of the "year from hell" and new beginnings. I know saying "it's over" is dangerous, because what if it isn't? But I guess I need to be ready to live with that uncertainty if I'm going to turn the page. The Greek islands beckon.

Thanks to so many of you who have been there for me and helped me get through this time in so many ways. With your love, I feel blessed.

Be well. Carpe diem.
Love, Tamara

Reflections

MAGIC HANDS: COMPLEMENTARY THERAPY FOR HEALING

While I was delighted with the results of my cataract surgery, the thrill of being able to see again was tempered by the shingles pain raging through the nerves that ran from my left hip down through my leg and into my foot. The pain would shift, darting from one part of my limb to another, but wherever it was it was constant and debilitating, especially after I fell. I tried everything to deal with it: physiotherapy, acupuncture, shots of vitamin B12, geranium oil. In desperation, I asked Dr. Verma for help. He gamely referred me to the pain clinic at the hospital, but there was a month-long waiting list to get a first appointment. I tried the drug for nerve pain he prescribed, but I was still hurting badly.

I hadn't had a massage since early March. Now that I'd healed from surgery, and radiation was over, massage for lymphatic drainage was highly recommended. It could improve the function of my lymphatic system following the removal of eighteen lymph nodes from my underarm and help stave off the dreaded lymphedema. I needed a massage therapist who had specialized training in lymphatic drainage and who could also work on my scar tissue to reduce the adhesions and keep my skin supple. Leesa recommended Amber at her clinic.

Lymphatic drainage, however, was far down on my list when I arrived at Amber's treatment room. I was desperate. After she had taken my health history, I told her, "I was looking for help with lymphatic drainage, but my main issue now is the terrible pain in my leg that's keeping me awake at night. It's driving me mad."

Amber took a deep breath, rolled up her sleeves and rubbed oil into her hands. I think she knew she had her work cut out for her and that this would be far from a relaxation massage. As I lay under the sheet on her table, she started to work her magic on my legs. She massaged not just the painful left leg but the right one too, working on the rest of my body, finding trigger points and releasing the pressure in my legs, hips, neck, and shoulders. There wasn't an inch of me that Amber didn't work on. With just an hour of intense massage, the nerve pain in my leg had quieted, significantly diminished for the first time since shingles had set in.

After another massage a few days later, my pain was miraculously gone. I was grateful to Amber, a talented young therapist who combines her considerable skill with a keen intuition about the body. She helped get me through a difficult time, and she continues to work with me on lymphatic drainage, my scar tissue, and therapeutic massage.

I also went back to Mark, my chiropractor of many years, who I'd been seeing preventively for spinal adjustments every few weeks until my surgery. Along with Leesa and now Amber, Mark was an important member of my complementary therapy team. Each had unique skills, talents, and approaches, sharing a focus on ways to nurture and encourage the body's innate ability to heal itself. I looked forward to continuing to work with them as I moved into recovery mode.

AN EVOLUTION OF SUPPORT:
FROM BOSOM BUDDIES TO BREAST FRIENDS

Once the pain finally abated, I could start to think about venturing outside the confines of my house and yard. I still needed a nap every afternoon, but I'd had enough of being reclusive. I was through with treatment and complications, and I was sleeping better and driving again. It was July and the weather was good. Now, it was a question of finding ways to get stronger and to build up my energy and stamina. It felt tentatively possible to face the world.

I was anxious to get to the monthly lunch with my "bosom buddies" in mid-July. I had missed the last couple of encounters, but it didn't matter. Everyone understood that not showing up was part of the ups and downs of what each of us was going through at one time or another.

There were warm hugs and greetings as we arrived at the restaurant, and as always, observations on each other's hair. The state of our hair at any given time reflected where we were in our chemo treatment or how far past chemo we had come. Most of the wigs were gone by now, a sign of both the return of our hair and the arrival of summer, because it was hot and sticky to wear a wig in the heat. My hair was about an inch long at that point, and it was coming in softer and curlier than before. It wasn't nearly as thick or as coarse as it had been, but I was at peace with the new look, glad to no longer be bald and curious to watch it unfold. A few of the women thought my hair looked good because it was relatively thick, but it was only because I'd had so much of it to start with. Little did I know that the wiry, uncontrollable hair I'd once tried to beat into submission had been an insurance policy that was now serving me well!

We sat squeezed into a circular booth, eating and listening intently as each of us shared our stories. I told them about my complications from radiation, my trips to emergency, my time in hospital, and about my ordeals with shingles and cataract surgery. Many of them were on one of the drugs that inhibit the production of estrogen to help prevent a return of cancer. With the ever-present fear of recurrence and wanting to do whatever they could to prevent it, they recounted the side effects they were experiencing, especially menopause-like symptoms such as hot flashes, joint pain, and leg cramps. Jane said "Just let me get to five years," referring to the benchmark for survival. I was the only one there not on an estrogen-inhibiting drug because my cancer isn't fed by estrogen or other hormones. I said I was worried about there being no drug I could take, but that I was working with Leesa to strengthen my immune system. I hoped it would stave off a recurrence without the side effects. Five years felt like an eternity.

Some of the women, especially the younger ones, were planning to go back to work. Some were looking forward to getting back to what they felt was their "normal" life, while others anticipated work with anxiety and dread. I found myself thinking that if I had to go back to work now, I'd probably crash. I was glad to have been at the lunch, but I was spent. I went home and lay down for a nap.

When we met again in the fall, our numbers had dwindled because many of the women were back at work and no longer available for two-hour lunches. At lunch that day, we figured we had to come up with a new formula for getting together. As there were several of us in our fifties and sixties who were not heading back to work, at least immediately, we decided to switch to monthly breakfasts. Gwen came up with a new name and "Breast Friends" was born.

Along the way, we collected three new Breast Friends, bringing our number to nine. With each new arrival into the circle, there was an easy connection, a welcoming into the sisterhood and a sharing of the joys and hardships of our lives. When things were rough for one of us, we tried to figure out how we could best offer our love and support. In the meantime, we eagerly anticipated coming together for the camaraderie, laughter, and the unique understanding of our shared experience.

As time went on, the conversation and tone within the group subtly began to shift. We were getting on with our lives in different ways – traveling, pursuing artistic ventures, embarking on new fitness routines, and a couple of us were going back to work full- or part-time. We heard about each other's art exhibitions, curling competitions, writing projects, retirement plans, far-off voyages, and adventures with children and grandchildren. We still talked about our breast cancer experiences, the aftermath, and our worries about recurrence, consulting each other about drugs, side effects, lymphedema, and follow-up with our doctors. But cancer was no longer the central focus. While it was the underpinning of our connection, most of us were now solidly on the road to recovery.

Here is a glimpse of a Breast Friends conversation that took place almost two years after most of us had finished treatment.

Jane: I wondered last night whether to come this morning. I thought, Maybe I don't need them anymore. Then I thought No, I'm not ready for that. I have to go.

Claudia: We have a connection and a bond.

Jane: The truth is, this group has moved on and we're growing together. You don't have to explain.

Kae: I wonder, are there groups that maintain the drama long past the time one needs to? I've heard them called "cancer cheerleaders," people who relive the drama ten years down the road. Is it a way of keeping it going because it was a time in people's lives when there was a lot of support and understanding that's no longer there?

Gwen: I've read that women with breast cancer do better in terms of survival if they join a support group. It's been two years for me, but the fear of it coming back is there. It's part of you. I don't think you can actually let go of it 100 percent. I've got a piece of myself prepared to face it, but in no way do I think my kids are okay with it.

Tamara: How do we contain that fear, keep it from infiltrating everything? We have to find ways to keep it in check.

Kae: Well, maybe it's being part of an honest group.

Gwen: I think we're pretty honest. I don't even have to talk about it here. It's just being with other women who really get it.

Kae: There was a time I felt resentful, when my family felt

I should have moved on a little faster. I was thinking Holy cow, give me a break. I'm talking to you about it *because* you're my family. Come on!

Jane: My son had just turned twenty when I sat him down for the talk. He said, "But you caught it early, Mom." I said, "Well, yes," and he said, "Then it's just an inconvenience."

Gwen: He knew it would probably comfort his mom.

Jane: My daughter reacted differently.

Kae: I think they all wanted to hear it was something that was going to be dealt with quickly. I found it hard to be on the reassuring end for them sometimes. I'd say "Yes, I think they've caught it early. I'm very optimistic, blah, blah, blah." But inside, I was absolutely freaking terrified.

Tamara: We're so used to taking care of them.

Kae: A good thing about a group like this is that we can share that honestly. I love coming to the group and seeing everyone looking so well!

Tamara: Isn't it fabulous? Look at us, every last one of us.

Kae: I bet we're not talking a lot about this outside of the group.

Gwen: No, I never talk to anybody about this.

Pat: The truth is that I don't really want to talk about it all the time. I want to just go on with my life, and live it as best, as joyfully, and as fully as I can each day.

Kae: Another reason I love the group is because we all seem to understand that there's a stage for recovery.

Tamara: Thankfully we're all still here. I can't imagine what would happen if something had happened to one of us. Pat, I truly believe what you're saying about "I want to find joy, I want to create, I want to live my life to the fullest." Do you think we're more driven to do those things because of what we've been through?

Recently, the Breast Friends were at breakfast, talking intently as we always do interspersed by moments of uproarious laughter. At one point, a woman none of us knew came over to our table and in a serious voice said, "I'm warning you that someone has just called the office in charge of the laughter bylaw to report you." We proceeded to break out into gales of laughter all over again, telling the woman we were a breast cancer support group. Then Claudia asked her, "Guess how many breasts there are around this table?" Shaking her head in disbelief, she shrugged her shoulders. We told her there were four breasts among the six of us. Momentarily subdued, we realized how grateful we all are for the group and what it means to us.

QUALITY OF LIFE DECISION: WORKING IT OUT
As my strength started to creep back, I wondered whether I would ever get to the point of being strong enough to go back to work. I thought about what my life had been like when I was working.

I loved my job in labor education, where I developed workshops and courses on a wide range of topics from collective bargaining to conflict resolution. I revelled in the challenge of making often complex material accessible and in creating rich learning experiences for the workers who came to our programs. I also enjoyed being in the classroom where I had the chance to experience the excitement of the participants learning from the courses and from each other.

But in truth, my job had too often consumed me. There was always too much work, not enough people to do it, and no organizational boundaries to contain it. It fed into my inclination to take on too much and to overextend myself because I believed in the work. While I enjoyed working with some of my colleagues who were often kindred spirits, the work environment was nonetheless stressful and demanding.

Too often I'd bring home the dregs, spent and overwhelmed by fatigue. When Larry retired, we made a deal. He would do his woodworking, take care of the house, do groceries, and make supper during the week. I would go to work and shop and cook on weekends. With no plans to retire for a few more years, the plan seemed reasonable enough. While it was probably my early morning workouts and my walking routine that kept me going, it often meant that I used the extra time not to relax, read, or see friends, but to do more work. On weekends, I would scramble to see my parents and friends and zone out to music as I made steaming pots of soup and took naps.

What would it be like to go back after going through cancer? Was it even possible? If I did return, what toll would it take on my health? When I pointedly asked Dr. Verma about it, he told me the chances of my cancer coming back were one in four. The odds were in my favor, but there were still significant dangers. I'd have to do my part to keep the 25 percent wolf at bay. What role could stress and depleted energy play?

I was still collecting long-term disability (LTD) and my extended health benefits were intact. With Larry on a fixed pension, our money situation was tight but manageable. How long would my LTD last? What if LTD cut me off? My head was spinning with all the questions, but I knew I was racing ahead of myself. How could the question be anything but moot in light of my current health situation and my compromised energy?

At the same time, I knew of far too many women who were facing financial pressures or lacked support from their employers. They'd gone back to work too soon after a serious illness and were paying a price with their mental and physical health. When a friend suggested I consider asking for a year's leave of absence without pay when my LTD ran out, my eyes lit up. Maybe that was a way to keep my options open. While we'd have to figure out the finances, it would also give my body the time it needed to heal, and I could see whether and to what extent it would recover. I put that idea under my hat to ponder further.

PRIVILEGE

I know my situation involved relative privilege as a white, reasonably well-educated, middle-class, married, heterosexual, Canadian-born woman. I live in Ottawa, Canada's capital city of about a million people with excellent health and cancer care services, all situated within a fifteen-minute drive from my house. These services are on a par with the best in the country, and operate within a highly regarded, publicly funded health care system.

Literate and English-speaking, I had a job with a good salary and extended health benefits. I was also included under Larry's extended health benefits with coverage for drugs as well as for certain aspects of complementary medicine, including naturopathic care, massage therapy, and chiropractic care. Although I had worked in temporary positions in the labor movement for almost twenty years, my situation had changed two years before my diagnosis when I got a permanent job in my workplace. This meant that I was covered by long-term disability insurance when I was not well enough to work. I also had a good job to return to, if and when I got well.

I had been married for almost thirty years and was in a mostly healthy and stable relationship, and our kids were now young adults. Our mortgage was paid off, we were virtually debt-free, and, although my income was substantially reduced during the course of my illness, we had enough money. I was fortunate to have good emotional and practical support from my family and friends.

What did all this mean? In addition to my material circumstances, I know it also shaped how I perceived and felt about myself and my place in the world. For example, I firmly believed I was entitled to receive the best health care possible, and was prepared to fight for it if I had to. I was determined not be a patient who would simply say "Yes, doctor" if I felt what he or she was proposing was questionable or not in my best interests. I had skills that proved useful during the course of my journey through cancer. I could speak up for myself when necessary and I could write.

My situation of relative privilege, however, couldn't keep me from the pitfalls that befall all who get cancer. Cancer is a great equalizer. No amount of privilege could keep me from falling into an abyss when I got my diagnosis, quaking in my boots when I felt awful during chemo, or from being terrified of dying before my time. But it did mean there were a number of significant areas that I didn't have to worry about on top of the other pressures and stresses I was dealing with.

In North America, breast cancer is sometimes known as a "white woman's disease," and the belief is that more Caucasian women are diagnosed with breast cancer than women of other racial and ethnic backgrounds. But it appears that immigrant women and women from ethnic minorities are less likely to be screened and thus don't get the benefits of early detection and treatment. This means that when they finally see a doctor, their disease is more advanced and the outcome less hopeful.

Dr. Angel Arnaout: Because the breasts are a private part of a woman's body, it's not something they want to share with other people in many parts of the world. Often, the physicians are male, so not only does the patient feel shame at what is happening to her body, but she may worry about having to go to a male physician.

Linda Corsini, the social worker at the Women's Breast Health Centre, described some of the women she counsels who are dealing with their breast cancer diagnosis in addition to a myriad of other issues.

Some of the women

- are visitors or recent arrivals in Canada and have not been in the country long enough to be covered by provincial health insurance plans

- are immigrant women who have been here longer and are covered by health insurance but still may have difficulty with 1) understanding how Canadian systems work, including health care, and 2) speaking, understanding, reading, and writing English or French

- may not have a family doctor

- have financial worries because they are not in the paid workforce, their family income is insufficient, or they are in low-paying jobs without drug plans, benefits, sick leave, or job security

- have young children and feel they can't cope with caring for them

- have a history of multiple and/or chronic health problems

- live hours away from the hospital and have to arrange for transportation and/or alternative living arrangements for some or all aspects of their care and treatment

- are isolated or live in relationships that are abusive or where there is little emotional or practical support, or where they fear being rejected or abandoned by their partners following the loss of a breast and the subsequent disfigurement

- wouldn't come to a support group because it's too complicated to find child care or transportation, because they live too far away, or because it is considered a cultural taboo in their community to reveal they have breast cancer in any kind of public way

- are terrified to take the first step.

Dr. Shailendra Verma: The questions of race, ethnicity and socio-economic status in relation to breast cancer are highly complex. White women are far more likely to go for screening for breast cancer. At the same time, the number of women of Chinese, East Asian, African, and Caribbean extraction with breast cancer has risen dramatically. That's who you'll see in the oncology ward, usually with very advanced breast cancers. They are often timid women who have never taken a stand in their lives or ethnic women who are sidelined and marginalized. What is this kind of woman going to do when she finds her breast cancer? She's going to get on with her life, which doesn't necessarily include going to the doctor. We need to find ways to reach out to her.

Who gets breast cancer? Why? Who gets screened regularly? Who doesn't? Who gets the benefit of early detection and treatment? Who doesn't? Why not? What can be done to prevent, screen for, and treat breast cancer in more equitable and inclusive ways that are attuned to the realities and diversity of our communities?

CHAPTER TEN

Recovery:
Rites of Passage

We bought tickets to Greece in April after Larry's prostate surgery, with a departure date set for mid-September. We would have just over three weeks there, spending a few days in Athens before heading to the islands. At the time, it was an act of faith to think we might make it, but we'd decided to keep our eyes on the prize I'd set my sights on many months before.

Greece marked a turning point in my journey with cancer. When we boarded the plane, I was excited about the adventure but shaky because I didn't know how my body would hold up. There would be lots of unknowns as we had deliberately not worked out the fine details of the trip, shades of post-chemo Mexico. While the last six months had included difficult times, the summer had been a time of healing. Greece was both a celebration and a test of my capacity and endurance, my first rite of passage into recovery.

After Greece, my recovery continued. I started thinking about what resuming my life might look like for the first time since my diagnosis. Although I wasn't sure what that would mean, I knew it would have to involve building up my strength and stamina. Since the complications from radiation and the bout of shingles, my muscles were still weak and I tired easily. I'd have to start slowly, but I was determined to get back to the Y and to start walking again with Denise in the mornings.

It was also time for a ritual of gratitude and celebration. When Larry and I were on Paros, we talked about the idea of hosting a "thank you" party. We weren't quite sure how we would do it, but we decided to collect a few handfuls of smooth stones when we were exploring the beaches. We were thinking they would be good tokens to offer the friends who had supported us throughout the journey. On the ferry back to Piraeus where we would spend our last night before flying home, I scribbled a poem of thanks to include with each stone.

In early December, we hosted our *Ef Charisto* ("thank you" in Greek) party. It was a celebration that was both poignant and jubilant, with great food, wine, music, and spirit. At one point, we gathered in the living room and I read my poem aloud. Then I invited everyone to take a card printed with the poem and choose a stone. Missy sang some of our favorite songs and played her guitar, and as the sun waned, some of us joined in with our own guitars, singing into the night.

✉ Healing Journey #10

November 14, 2010

Dear friends and family,

I spent the last few weeks of summer at the cottage, healing my body and spirit in the soothing waters of Marble Lake and in the woods around me, glad to be getting stronger and to be reading again after the dark days with my cataract. Larry and I had good visits with friends from out of town who came to spend time with us there, and it was fun to have Labour Day weekend with Rachel, Daniel, and Eric. Slowly, my life force, which I feared might be gone for good during the bleak days of hospitalization, shingles, visual impairment, weakness, and pain, was coming back. I was starting to believe that my body might be capable of healing and being well again.

One of my big challenges continues to be to keep the fear of my cancer recurring in check, to acknowledge that it could happen but to avoid obsessing about it. Being "triple negative," (estrogen and progesterone receptor negative as well as HR2 negative), means that the drugs that often follow active breast cancer treatment to block the effects of hormones on breast tissue are not effective in my case. Soon after I got out of hospital, I started doing IVC again, this time preventively. In the IVC room, we arrive as strangers who come to know intimate details about each other in no time. Tethered to our IV poles, we are also tethered to the hope that the vitamin C running through our veins will help fight our cancer, reduce the side effects of treatment, or prevent a recurrence.

There is always anxiety when one of the regulars goes missing from the IVC room. I noticed that Najah hadn't been there for a few weeks, and at my weekly session mid-August, I learned she had died the previous weekend at forty-nine. Najah had been diagnosed two years before with cancer in her breast that was of unknown origin (this happens in about 10 percent of cancers). She underwent treatment and thought she had beaten it, but it came back with a vengeance in her lungs and bones in January, when her doctor gave her nine months to live. She seemed to be doing okay until July when it entered her brain.

A few weeks before she died, Najah and I were alone in the IVC room. We wept as she asked why she had to go so soon and why her family had to go through the anguish of losing her. She wondered how she would cope with the excruciating pain of dying. When I heard she was gone, I was unspeakably sad. I hoped that her pain hadn't been unbearable. Thankfully, it hadn't lasted long.

As the first hint of fall sweetened the air, it was time to prepare for our long dreamed of (but hardly dared hoped for) departure for Greece. We had decided to do minimal planning for our time there. We booked three days in Athens and three days on one of the islands, then we'd follow our hearts and noses for the rest of our three weeks. Friends helped us decide that Naxos, an island in the Cyclades with which they've had a long love affair, would be a good destination.

I was strangely relaxed leading up to our departure, so unlike my usual frantic self before traveling. It was good to have planned a quiet weekend before leaving, allowing for a new kind of "spaciousness," as Joyce would say, to set in. The uncluttered time let me move more slowly and thoughtfully, thinking about what I needed to take instead of packing too much, remembering things I might have forgotten otherwise, like the 1000 euros I had stashed away in a wallet I wasn't taking. I was calm and excited at the same time. I was excited about going to Greece for symbolic reasons to mark the end of my year of treatment and complications. It was also because I'd never been to Greece but had wanted to go, especially to the islands, for such a long time. While I wasn't busting to leave town, I was glad to be well enough to go on this adventure.

It was hard to believe that so much had changed for the better.

When I'd imagined Greece as the "prize" a year ago, it was a pipe dream. Would I be alive a year later? If I were alive, would I be in any shape to travel? We had cancelled plans to go to Niagara-on-the-Lake and Blue Skies over the summer because they would have been physically and otherwise impossible. Yet here I was going off to Greece, hoping against hope that my newfound energy and stamina would endure.

A neighbor drove us to the airport and sent us off on our flights, first to Montreal and then to Athens. I couldn't figure out why the attendant on the first leg of the trip was smiling at me throughout the flight. But as we were about to file out of the plane, she told me she had noticed the compression sleeve I was wearing to prevent lymphedema, which can be induced by the air pressure on long flights. She was just back to work after eighteen months off with breast cancer. We bonded instantly, and I went on to Athens knowing the sisterhood was alive and well.

Other than the pickpocket who slid a wad of euros out of Larry's jeans in the crowded metro on our first day in Athens, we found the Greeks friendly and helpful. We loved wandering the streets, ogling the markets and climbing up to the Acropolis looking over the city, the weather sunny and warm but not too hot, the food fresh and delicious. After three whirlwind days in Athens, we took a five-hour ferry ride to Naxos, where the goddess must have been with me because I didn't get seasick!

We stayed in an eight-room hotel on the beach at Mikri Vigla, which means "look-out" because the people there were always on the watch for pirates. We ate breakfast on our balcony looking out over the sea and headed to a *taverna* nearby for supper. It would be easy to live on a 100-mile diet on the bounty of Naxos: fruit and vegetables of all kinds, fresh olives, wine, fish and seafood, lamb, creamy yogurt, and feta.

After the first few way too busy days, we got our bearings and figured out a good rhythm. We'd head for the bakery in the morning for warm fresh bread and pastries for breakfast, then swim, read, and hang out at the pool and the beach till mid-afternoon. Then we'd go off on an adventure to discover a new village, beach, or ruin, coming back to nap before going to find supper.

I loved visiting the temple of Demeter, goddess of the harvest, where the ancients made sacrifices for a bountiful crop surrounded by rolling terraced fields, olive groves, vineyards, and pastures dotted with sheep and goats. Zeus is said to have grown up on Naxos, and Mt. Zeus rises up in the middle of the island, so it was easy to imagine Zeus striking out with his thunderbolt on the night we had a thunderstorm.

Some days, we wended our way up steep mountainsides in our rented sub-compact on narrow, zigzagging roads with hairpin turns and views of the island that took our breath away. We came upon tiny mountain villages that date back over a thousand years when the people fled to the mountains to get away from the ever-menacing pirates. Apiranthos, my favorite, is carved into the mountainside, with ancient white stone houses and narrow marble streets accessible only by foot or donkey. An Apiranthos native, Manilos Glezos, was the celebrated resistance fighter who replaced the Nazi flag with the Greek flag on top of the Acropolis during WWII.

The villagers were friendly as they went about their day, sweeping, washing, shlepping, sitting in outdoor cafes and tavernas. I loved watching the locals, their faces and hands so expressive it didn't matter that I didn't understand. My few Greek words were pathetic, but people seemed to appreciate the effort. It was fun to think about the Greek roots of so many English words: *philo, polis, sophia, logos, psyche, eros*, etc. So many of our big ideas come from Greek!

The beaches of Naxos are beautiful, the sea a mesmerizing azure against whitewashed houses, with hot pink or red hibiscus or bougainvillea cascading down the sun-bleached walls. I got plenty of exercise, swimming three times a day, and I started to feel more like my old self. Sometimes I even forgot I'd had cancer, then I'd remember how hard it had been, which made it seem like a miracle that I was in Greece and in one piece.

Keen to see another island, we took the ferry to nearby Paros. I loved the scooter we rented there. I'd forgotten how great it is to experience the exhilarating ride with all your senses, smelling the wild mountain thyme, breathing the salt air, like being on a bicycle without the work! We explored beaches and mountain villages, ending up back at the hotel pool by mid-afternoon to read, swim, play Upwords, nap, then walk to the village for a fabulous supper. The Greeks eat late, often not until 8 or 9 p.m. or even later, which makes sense because they take siestas. So sane and healthy!

On Day 2 with the scooter, we were touring the coastline of Paros, heading into the village of Piso Livadi. Not sure of our directions, we were slowly approaching a stop sign when we hit a patch of gravel and spilled over. It happened almost in slow motion, but there we were, stunned, pinned to the ground under the scooter. Within seconds, a local pulled up and rushed over to see if we were okay. Shaken, we set the scooter upright and assessed the damage. I only had a scraped knee, but Larry had taken the brunt of the impact and had pain around his ribcage. Thankfully, we were able to get back in the saddle and ride to Naoussa.

It was strange to be lying on the ground, thinking about what a bizarre twist of fate it was to have come all this way after the year from hell and then have a scooter accident. The goddess must have been with us again because we were lucky, all things considered. Larry resisted getting checked out until a couple of days later, when still in pain, he decided to make sure there were no broken ribs or a punctured lung.

The next morning, we took the bus to the hospital in Perikia. There, we waited five minutes in emergency, where a doctor checked Larry's lungs and sent him down the hall for an X-ray, which was taken right away. Larry took the X-ray back to the doctor who said it looked fine, but that the bruising could last a week or so. The whole process took less than twenty minutes, after which we were sent off with the X-ray and a prescription for painkillers, all at no charge. It was a glimpse of what might be a great model for health care, but we had to wonder if the lack of fees for tourists was contributing to the Greek economic crisis!

Larry needed to lie low for a bit, so we turned in the scooter and arranged to rent a car for our last two days to explore a bit more of Paros. In the meantime, Larry rested, read, and healed, I swam, walked, and explored, and, of course, we played many games of Upwords. In spite of the mishap, we left Paros and Greece elated.

It was good to come home to a taste of fall, with some color still left on the trees. I had long visits with my mom, and went back to the Y for the first time since I had crashed in May, swimming, doing cardio and weights tentatively at first, then slowly building up the time and intensity of my workouts. Denise and I started walking again in the early mornings, and she convinced me to take a Nordic pole walking class with her at the community center.

Rachel had given me a mother/daughter weekend for my birthday last April, but it couldn't happen till November because of my health. When the appointed weekend arrived, it was fun to finally board the train and head for Montreal. It was a workday for Rachel so I'd planned to have lunch with Monique, who had retired last year to her home town of Sorel, both of us looking forward to hearing more about the changes in our lives. I took the Metro to Mont Royal and walked up to Rachel's third-floor flat to leave my bag, then walked over to Les Folies to find Monique.

We ate, locked in conversation about cancer, retirement, Paros, kids, love, food, letting go, finding centeredness, learning to follow our hearts at this time of our lives, etc. After three solid hours, Monique came with me to buy a winter coat at a great price before we had big hugs and a heartfelt "*à la prochaine.*"

I was anxious to savor the flavors of Greece again with Rachel, so we had supper at a Greek restaurant on Rue St Denis that night.

Rachel's roommate was jamming with a friend when we got back to their place; it was fun to listen and sing along. The next day we walked to the old port, saw a film, hit a spa, came home for naps, then went off to a Peruvian "bring your own wine" family restaurant a few blocks away. On Sunday morning, we worked out at Rachel's gym, hung out, and wandered through the Plateau. As we watched life on the street from the balcony waiting for my ride home, we mused about how much fun we'd had with hardly any plans, vowing to do it again soon.

Back in Ottawa, I met an old friend at a concert after not seeing her for ages, so she hadn't known about my cancer. She suggested we have lunch on Remembrance Day as she'd be off work. At lunch, she was keen to hear the story of my year from hell. I knew telling her would be different than when I was with people I see regularly or who read my Healing Journey letters, because they've been with me along the way and with them I don't have to start at the beginning.

I found myself trembling as I recounted my angst and fear following the diagnosis, the "lucky" infection that got me on track for treatment, the paradox of chemo, finding the dream team of doctors, the complications, pain, weakness, etc. I also told her about the silver linings and the love and support that had flowed, often in unexpected ways. I said I felt like I had been to war and how strange it was to return to the so-called normal world so irrevocably altered, wondering whether anyone could understand where I'd been. We mused about how the language of cancer is often bellicose: cancer "invades" our bodies, we "combat" the disease, we strive to "conquer" it, we die after a "valiant battle." If we make it we are "survivors," if not we have "lost the battle."

We talked about the complicated symbolism of both poppies (lest we forget/glory of war/peace) and pink ribbons (remembering the women who have died/the cure/"pinkwashing" – companies whose products pollute and damage our bodies that direct a tiny portion of their profits to finding a cure for breast cancer). The fear, the losses, and the hopes: what we're supposed to think about on

Remembrance Day seems so narrow. There are so many other wars to remember.

I am also remembering how important you have all been to me over the last fifteen months.

Be well. Carpe diem.
Love, Tamara

Reflections

KEEPING FEAR IN CHECK

I was conscious of trying to keep my fears of a recurrence in check: fears of the remnants of cancer spreading to one of my organs or my bones, of going through treatment and having to face the prospect of dying before my time all over again. I think it's true that the longer the time that has passed since my diagnosis and the farther away I am from being "inside" the treatment experience, the more able I am to quiet my fears. But it's also true that the fears will never go away. Fear is simply an ongoing reality. Like every other cancer patient, I will always live with it.

Because of my triple negative status, I was being monitored more closely than usual, which meant I was still seeing Drs. Verma, Meng, or Arnaout every four months. Sometimes when I saw Dr. Verma, he had lots of time for me. He was attentive, warm, and caring. At other times, he seemed more rushed. I realized after a few such appointments that this was the way he managed his triage system. It made sense that he would devote more time to the patients who needed him most at any particular time. If he was in a hurry and I had more questions than he had time for that day, he would smile broadly, look me straight in the eye, and say, "But you're not complicated!" as he prepared to take flight. I surmised that this meant I hadn't made the cut as a patient who required his undivided attention that day. Ever conscious that I too had once been complicated, I was relieved to now be less so. While I wished it could be otherwise, I appreciated how Dr. Verma justly meted out the time he spent with his patients on the basis of our respective needs. I was no longer as needy.

Dr. Shailendra Verma: It's good for me to learn that even the uncomplicated patient feels complicated.

Once my post-surgery pathology report showed the cancer was gone, I was anxious to get my portocath removed. It didn't bother me physically, although I had to have it flushed at the chemo room each month. But its presence was symbolic. When I asked Dr. Verma, he said he wanted to leave it in for another year, just in case.

It was sobering to realize that he didn't want me to have to go through the surgical insertion process again if my cancer came back, so he understandably was erring on the side of caution. I'm sure it was a wise decision, soundly based on his decades of experience, his knowledge of the statistics on recurrence, and his mindfulness of the need to spend health care dollars judiciously. But for me, deciding to detach the portocath and then extract it from my body would have been an act of faith and a powerful symbol of victory. Our victory, Dr. Verma's and mine. It would also have gone a long way toward quelling my fears of becoming complicated again.

Dr. Meng says keeping the portocath for a year is standard practice. She also says it's important to pay attention to any headaches, coughing, or pain that come along, otherwise regular things that could indicate a possible recurrence. They will monitor me closely with check-ups, blood tests, mammograms, MRIs. I carry on working with Leesa, taking supplements and doing intravenous vitamin C preventively. So living with and beyond cancer presents yet another paradox. How do I carry on with my life in a hopeful way without obsessing about the possibility of a recurrence?

Dr. Leesa Kirchner: Support to prevent recurrence is not generally a focus of mainstream oncology. Once you're out of treatment, the message is too often, "Good-bye. We'll do scans, and if and when it comes back, we'll treat you again." I find people are sometimes more upset about the fear of recurrence than by their initial diagnosis. I see so much frustration and shock at that time. When they come in and I say, "There are things we can do to help reduce the risk of recurrence," I see tears coming down just because we're having the conversation. They're relieved to know they can actually do something proactive to help prevent a recurrence. That kind of empowerment is a big thing.

Nadia, a woman in her early thirties in my support group, has just been through a recurrence of an aggressive breast cancer. She's had a rough time but is coming out the other side. At a recent Breast Friends breakfast, she told us about a reptile exhibit at a fundraising event she'd recently attended to celebrate people living with cancer. Nadia had always been terrified of snakes, but she decided that this time she was going to try to touch the large anaconda coiled in the keeper's arms. But when she stepped forward to touch it, she realized she was no longer afraid. After going through two cancers, two regimens of treatment, and coming face to face with her mortality, her other fears, including her fear of snakes, disappeared.

What about the fears our families experience? How do our spouses, children, parents, siblings cope with their fears? It was a question that had plagued me throughout the previous year. One night on Naxos, Larry and I had supper at a taverna in the countryside. We were relaxed and had fallen in love with Greece and with each other all over again.

There was a pressing question I'd needed to ask Larry for a long time. I had to know what living with me through cancer had been like for *him*, now that I was out of the woods and feeling so much better, now that we were in Greece, having a great time together, and enjoying a delicious meal.

We were about halfway through the meal when I posed the question as gently as I could, "Were you scared you were going to lose me?" I asked tentatively, watching Larry's face, hoping we could finally have that conversation.

Larry looked away. Finally, he spoke. "Of course it was always there in my head, the worry you might not make it, the fear of losing you, thinking about what life would be like for me and the kids without you. But I tried to focus my energy on giving you what you needed to get through treatment, to be the one you could lean on." He went on, "I always felt like we were going through it together. But

I had to create boundaries to make sure everything in our lives didn't get overwhelmed by the cancer experience, to deal with it in a way that made sense for me."

He took a deep breath. "I used to go crazy on the nights before you'd have chemo, worrying about how hard it was going to be for you. I tried to put myself in your shoes. I was always asking questions and thinking about different scenarios so we could come up with the best strategy for fighting the cancer. I know I wasn't always able to give you what you needed emotionally. But I did worry. I did suffer along with you. It was inevitable that I had to deal with the possibility that I could lose you. Thankfully, what I hoped for won out."

I was relieved to have him express his fears out loud for the first time. I reached out for his hands as the waiter brought dessert over to our table, an amazing chocolate pastry, a lovely Greek tradition where the house offers a sweet ending to the evening.

COPING WITH LOSSES

How do we handle the losses of our sister patients, our partners in arms, who sat, walked, talked, infused, were in support groups, and communed with us side by side in countless ways? We mourn their deaths and lament the loss of what their lives might have been as we weep for the families left behind. We think of the times we shared as we try to make sense of why it was them and not us this time.

But besides mourning our friends, each loss is a threat that awakens the fear we harbor for our own lives. It wreaks havoc with our tenuous equilibrium, spilling seeds of fear from the sacks we carry on our backs as we return from the country of cancer.

At the time of my diagnosis, I had several friends who had survived the disease, but my friend Martha was the only one I knew personally who hadn't made it, one of the 5,100 women who die of breast cancer each year in Canada. Martha was dying of breast cancer when I was going through the tests that led to my diagnosis. She was fifty-nine when she died, just a year older than me.

Martha and I had a long history. We had met thirty years before when we were both in our twenties and had gone through our pregnancies and the births of our sons. Later, we helped each other plan the Bar Mitzvahs of our sometimes wayward boys. It was the kind of friendship where we'd come together intensely at various points, lose track of each other for extended periods, then rekindle our connection as if it had always been there.

Martha's quiet wisdom had deepened since her diagnosis eight years earlier. She had gone through remissions, recurrences, and endless rounds of treatment in the years that followed. Sometimes, she could carry on with her work as a talented museum curator; sometimes she'd have to go on extended periods of sick leave. In spite of the grim truth that her cancer had spread to her liver and bones, she fought it hard with everything she had, fervently hoping to see her two boys grow up.

Larry and I went to Martha's funeral. It was a beautiful service filled with haunting traditional melodies and memories, and I was glad to be there to remember her life in the company of her family and friends. But as I sat on the hard wooden bench still raw from my own diagnosis, I wondered how I dared hope to beat my cancer when Martha hadn't, and whether her fate awaited me too.

I thought of Martha often throughout my cancer journey. I wished I'd known then what I know now so I could have better understood what life was like for her, so I could have been a better friend. I missed Martha badly, but at times I'd feel her presence when I was going through chemo, when I was losing my hair, when I was worrying about my kids. She was gone but I still found comfort in her "company," believing she was rooting for me, urging me to live fully and well.

The odds are stacked against us; we lose people because of the company we keep – the Breast Friends, the patients in the IVC room at Leesa's clinic, all of whom have or had cancer. Najah would arrive at the IVC room sporting neon baseball caps and sexy halter tops. After spending hours together for weeks and months on end, the rest of us would get edgy and nervous when she or one of the other regulars didn't show up for a while. This was especially true if it was someone who was dealing with a deadly cancer, a metastasis, or a recurrence. We knew they probably weren't away on holidays. Najah, whose mysterious cancer had spread, was one of those in the room whom we came to know like family. They'd be with us and then, sometimes without warning, they'd be inexplicably gone, long before their time.

Sometimes, I'd only find out what had happened when I read the obituaries. Reading the obits was a habit I'd developed long before my cancer, but I now read them with new eyes, warily scanning the pages with a new urgency and dread. As the months wore on, I'd asked Leesa about my fellow patients who seemed to have "disappeared" from her clinic. I needed to know because it was an important part of facing the truth about my cancer. With eyes brimming, Leesa would shrug her shoulders helplessly and nod to confirm the death.

We were always careful about how we talked about it though, because some in the IVC crowd made it clear they didn't want to know. They found it too heartbreaking, too hard to take in on top of everything they were dealing with. It got in the way of hope. I tried to hold on to Joyce's advice to do all that I can to be well and accept the mystery.

Dr. Leesa Kirchner: Early on, I felt almost uncomfortable talking about death. I didn't know how to broach it, I never knew what to do. It's hard because you want to offer people hope. You don't want to be morbid, but you also have to be realistic. It's taken me a long time, but it has slowly changed. It's not something that you can learn. It's just something that has to happen.

THE NATURE OF "RECOVERY"

There was no doubt I was feeling a lot better. I was cancer free, I was several months past the end of treatment and complications, and I was not in pain. But it was exhausting even to think about going back to work. Instinctively, I knew my health was still fragile. What would it mean to add long hours, cross-country travel, and considerable stress to a beleaguered body that was just getting back on its feet?

At the same time, I felt that when I had abruptly left work following my diagnosis, I had left "broken." There was a part of me that wanted to go back to work duly healed, repaired, and "whole." I had hoped that when the time was right for me to retire, I'd be in a position to leave well.

When I saw Joyce, I told her I was preoccupied with finding a way to go back to work whole. As I sat on her blue couch sipping tea in her small home office, she looked straight at me. She asked, "After what you've been through, how will going back to work allow you to be well?"

My dilemma about recovery and my job soon came to a head when I received a phone call from the insurance company rep in charge of my long-term disability benefit file. From his point of view, the time was approaching for me to think about going back to work (and getting off benefits). What was my current health status? What were my plans? The insurance rep said he would assign a disability consultant to meet with me to discuss putting a plan in place for a graduated return to work. The idea was that if I went back to work part-time and incrementally increased to full-time over the two or three months, my chances of a successful return would be greater.

My employer also got in touch with me at around the same time. My position, now vacant for over a year, had not been filled. When the new director of education and I met for coffee, he told me what was happening in the department and outlined the projects he hoped I might take on. Naturally, he also wanted to know my thoughts about coming back to work. I told him I wasn't ready to go back to work yet, that my stamina wasn't anywhere near where it needed to be, and that I was still feeling fragile. Although disappointed, he seemed to hear what I was trying to say. He said he'd do whatever he could to support me.

When I talked to Leesa, she said she believed that with the aggressive cancer, treatment, and complications I'd been through, it was far too soon for me to even be thinking about it. She referred to the need for a period of recovery, the time when one is no longer sick and in treatment but not yet well either. When I asked how long that would be, she replied that it needed to be at least as long as the time spent undergoing treatment and dealing with complications. In my case, it added up to almost an additional year off. That would take me to the summer of 2011, now eight months away.

I knew if I wanted to extend my time off and keep my benefits, I'd need the support of my medical doctors. Leesa pointed out that sadly, a note from my naturopath wasn't likely to carry much weight with the insurance company. It would have to come from at least one of my specialists, but I had no idea how they would respond to my request for a letter.

My appointment with Dr. Verma happened first. He was pleased with my progress and how well I was doing, but he was not prepared to write the letter. He said he believed that the sooner I could get back to my regular life, including going back to work, the better it would be for my health and well-being.

Dr. Meng tuned in immediately to what I was saying about my low energy and stamina, the stress my job entailed, my fears of a recurrence, and what it would mean to go back to work too soon. She understood the value of what recovery time could offer me in the short and long term. When Dr. Meng and my family doctor each wrote a letter to the insurance company, my benefits were extended for another few months.

Dr. Joanne Meng: As physicians, we feel completely uncomfortable knowing how much time to give. We have had no training in this. I tend to be generous on how much time I'm willing to give. It's about so much more than the cancer.

Unfortunately, the concept of recovery is barely recognized. If it is acknowledged at all, it is too often seen as a luxury with few institutional supports and with only a small minority of workers able to afford to take the time they need. There are pressures all around us to pull ourselves together, to get back to work and return to our "normal" lives as soon as possible. It is too rare that this essential phase of our healing is taken into account in any meaningful way.

The pressures can come from insurance companies anxious to end our disability coverage, from employers who want us back on the job, or from doctors unwilling to sign the necessary forms to extend our leave. It can come from our families who may be dealing with the financial constraints caused by our not working or who are simply anxious for this time of illness to be over and for us to "get on with it." It can also come from us, from feeling guilty about taking too much time off and not pulling our financial weight at home.

It's complicated. We're no longer technically sick or in treatment. But while we may appear well, our bodies are still working hard to recover. We are still healing from a catastrophic illness that has wreaked havoc with every aspect of our physical and psychological being.

Recovery also connects to privilege. How many women can afford to take the "extra" time to recover? What happens if we go back to our traditional roles and domestic responsibilities before we're ready? If we worked in a low-wage job before we got sick, chances are we don't have long-term disability coverage or savings in the bank. Our employers are unlikely to hold our jobs for us beyond their legal requirement to do so. So we return to work both at home and in the workplace not sick *but not well either*, putting our health and ourselves at serious risk.

While most people can't afford to take time off to recover properly, the irony is that the more we and our employers invest in our recovery, the more it will pay off in terms of our health and productivity. When we return to work after taking sufficient time to heal and recover, we'll have more energy, resilience, and stamina. We'll be more productive with less chance of a relapse or recurrence.

CHAPTER ELEVEN

"To Life"
and the Future

When breast cancer befell me in 2009, I became a statistic, one of the 22,700 women diagnosed with breast cancer each year in Canada (according to the Canadian Cancer Society). Together, we are the size of a small city! We know that breast cancer is epidemic, killing more women than any other disease. One in eight women in Canada will go through it at some point in their lives.

Millions of dollars have been raised to support breast cancer research through the efforts of hundreds of thousands of generous people. These include many survivors who have walked, run, or donated to the Run for the Cure and the Pink Ribbon campaign.

While these efforts have raised awareness and accomplished a great deal, *Pink Ribbons, Inc.* by Samantha King (2006) and the National Film Board of Canada's 2011 documentary based on her book reveal the underbelly of the Pink Ribbon Campaign. They point to the corporations that continue to poison our increasingly toxic environment, all the while "pinkwashing" their guilt. The emphasis is on "the cure," rather than on prevention. As Dr. Susan Love, the esteemed American breast cancer specialist and activist, says in the film, "How can we find a cure for breast cancer if we don't know what causes it?"

> Dr. Shailendra Verma: I don't think we've discovered much more since I've been in oncology. With all these trillions of dollars that have gone into cancer research, I'm ashamed that we haven't been more collaborative about finding some of these real answers. We need more research to try to prevent women from getting breast cancer in the first place.

Although survival rates are improving, the irony is that the odds of getting breast cancer increase every year. While this is partly due to early detection with more effective screening, there seems little doubt that breast cancer is also more prevalent because of the rise in pollution and toxicity in so much of what we eat, drink, breathe and put on our faces, hair, and skin.

This reality is one of the many paradoxes I encountered as I traveled through the country of cancer.

I continue to be struck by how the entire experience of cancer is characterized by paradoxes. Right from the beginning during my first round of chemo when one nurse referred to my chemo drug as the *red devil* and another nurse later called it the *red angel*, the paradoxes continued to unfold in startling and sobering ways. For example:

- While I hated losing my hair, it was a sign that chemo was working.

- At the same time as I was striving to be the captain of my own ship, I had to accept that any control I thought I had over my life and my destiny was an illusion.

- As I was more able to accept and open up to others about my vulnerability, people responded with an abundance of love and caring, which in turn gave me strength.

- While I was disappointed to learn there was no drug available to help prevent a recurrence of my particular cancer, I was relieved not to have to deal with debilitating side effects.

- In the midst of cancer treatment, I learned what my survivor sisters meant by the gifts that would come my way, I could finally put myself front and center and seek out the spaciousness I had so long craved.

- While going through cancer was the loneliest time in my life, it was also the time when I felt the most loved and cared for.

- Once I could accept that dying "before my time" was a possible outcome of my cancer, I was less afraid and I could more fully embrace and fight for my life.

- When the future appeared murky, unpredictable, and illusive, I was finally able to live in the present.

My entire journey with breast cancer sent me crashing to rock bottom and forced me to confront the essence of who I was. It rattled and shook me to the core so completely that there was no possibility of returning to my old ways. Despite being battered and bruised, my hope is that I have come out better and wiser – the ultimate paradox.

✉ Healing Journey #11

June 28, 2011

Dear friends and family,

It's been a long time since my last Healing Journey letter, I know I've been remiss for not writing sooner. I've wanted to fill you in on what's been happening, but the truth is I've been struggling to figure out how writing fits into my life now, maybe because I've been feeling stronger. The funny thing is that I was probably a more disciplined writer when I was feeling crummy, at least in part because I wasn't able to do much else. I wonder if that's why there are so many writers who were invalids for significant periods of their lives. But the good news is that I've regained a good deal of my strength, there is lots going on in my life, and, thankfully, there are many more choices now.

I was exhilarated after our travels to the Greek islands last fall, where Larry and I went to celebrate the end of the year from hell. I continued to ride on the magic of our trip as I steadily gained in strength and started thinking about my life from now on. Then, a few days after sending out my last Healing Journey letter in November, I received a call from the hospital to schedule me for a CT scan. My heart sank, as I knew something must have shown up on the mammogram or chest X-ray I'd had recently, part of my post-treatment monitoring routine. When I called Dr. Verma's nurse to find out, she told me that an opacity, a shadow, had shown up on my left lung that hadn't been evident before. I asked if I should worry about it, and she said she wasn't going to tell me not to because I would anyway.

My lightness of spirit sank with the news. Had the cancer spread to my lung? Was this exuberant moment of my return to health about to be extinguished? Would I have to go through treatment all over again? Would I make it this time? I tried hard to be zen about it, but although there were lots of possible explanations for what had been found besides cancer (the remnants of an infection, scar tissue, etc.), the box in which I had packed away my fear of a recurrence had exploded.

The next day was November 16th, the first anniversary of my father's death. My mom, Larry, and I had made plans to go to "his" tree that day, the gorgeous Pacific maple where we had scattered his ashes. It was a poignant moment, even a bit awkward as we stood arm in arm in front of the stark, leafless tree on that damp morning, wondering what to do. My mom saved the day by suggesting we sing, and so we did, offering up some of the old songs my dad had loved: "Goodnight Irene," "We Shall not be Moved," and "Solidarity Forever."

Afterwards, my mom and I sat on a park bench, and I told her about the X-ray results. She listened, acknowledging my fears as she cautioned me not to race ahead of myself. Wise as always in a crisis, she pointed out that there was a good chance the results of the CT scan would turn out to be something other than cancer. If it was cancer, we would cross that bridge and figure out how to deal with it. After I drove my mom back to her place, I felt grateful for her love and wisdom, and wondered how I'd get through the next ten days of waiting and fretting, wishing I could go to sleep until it was over.

I had the CT scan a couple of days later, and was told the results would come in a week or so. We had planned a trip to Toronto, and were en route when I got the call saying the CT scan was clear, and as I got off the phone we let out cries of relief and jubilation. Elated but spent, I resolved to put my terror back in its box once again.

I was feeling pretty well, but I knew I was nowhere near being ready to go back to work. While there was much that I loved about being an education rep at the Canadian Labour Congress, I was exhausted thinking about what it would mean for my health if I went back to my intense and demanding job. How could I work full-time, flat out when my strength and stamina were still so limited and when I needed daily naps? Although I was cancer-free and beyond treatment and complications, I was in the in-between place of not being sick but not entirely well either. I knew in my gut that I needed to respect the recovery phase in which I now found myself. Honoring it would allow me the time and space to truly heal, in many ways as essential as going through treatment. With the support of my doctors, my long-term disability benefits were extended for a few more months.

My routine involved getting to the Y several mornings a week for cardio, weights, and stretching, and sometimes laps in the pool, and my LTD insurer got me involved in a rehab program with a physiotherapist to build my strength. Denise and I went for long morning walks along the canal, I joined a fabulous Yogathrive class for cancer patients and survivors, and I fell in love anew with cross-country skiing in the winter and cycling in the spring. I carried on seeing my "dream team" of doctors Verma, Meng, and Arnaout as well as my amazing complementary health care providers: Mark, my chiropractor, Amber, my massage therapist, and Joyce, my coach. I continued to work with Leesa, my naturopathic oncologist, to build up my immune system, which included receiving IVC once a week. I got together with my mom and with my friends when I could and napped in the late afternoon. I mostly laid low in the evening, when Larry and I would play Upwords, drink pots of green tea, and listen to music.

While my health steadily improved, there were difficult things happening to some of the people closest to me. Larry's health took a turn for the worse a few months ago, when the pain in his legs became constant, relentless, and debilitating. He's now in the process of seeing various specialists to figure out the cause and determine the next steps. When my friend Debbie was diagnosed with endo-metrial cancer last winter, we couldn't believe cancer had befallen both of us within the year. It's been hard to see her go through the terrors of diagnosis and the ravages of treatment, but I'm glad to be there for her, co-ordinating rides to her radiation treatments, bringing food, and getting together to sing with Missy.

When I finally had my portocath removed in April, it felt like I'd come full circle. I'd been ecstatic eighteen months earlier when it had been surgically inserted under the skin on my chest, because it was so much less cumbersome than the PICC line I'd started out with. Most importantly, it had allowed me to swim, and each swim had felt like an immersion in a ritual bath of healing. But once I was through treatment I wanted the portocath out. On each visit to Dr. Verma I'd ask if I could have it removed, and he'd say, "Let's wait until next time." That is, until he finally said "okay" at my appointment in April, fifteen months after finishing chemo.

I sat in the hospital waiting room, feeling light-hearted as I waited in glad anticipation for the minor surgery that would remove the portocath. A young woman, wan and scared, recently diagnosed with breast cancer, was there waiting anxiously to have hers inserted. I wanted to reassure her, to tell her she'd be able to swim with her portocath, and that I wished her strength and courage in the battles ahead. That I hoped she'd beat her cancer and be back soon to get her port out, and that she'd have the chance to come full circle too.

I turned sixty in April. It was a significant milestone by any count, but especially after doing battle with cancer. Not long before, I hadn't known if I'd make it to sixty. In the weeks and months leading up to my birthday, I found I wasn't worrying about gray hair and wrinkles, or even about the aches and pains of aging. Rather, I was looking forward to the journey of getting older not with dread but with yearning. I realized how I hoped to have the chance to get old. Turning sixty was an important step along the way, so it was great to be able to celebrate it with friends and family, to sing and toast l'chaim, "to life."

Turning sixty was also a time for making big decisions, such as whether to go back to work or not. I had been stewing about it for months, and had been all over the map in my deliberations. There was part of me that felt that when I had left work to go on sick leave I had been broken, and that it would be an important part of my healing for me to go back and to eventually leave well. I also had to consider the significant penalty I would take on my pension if I retired before age sixty-three.

At the same time, some of the burning questions that might have plagued me had I not been catapulted into cancer had diminished in importance. Who was I separate from my identity connected to my work? What would happen to the relationships I had developed through work? Would they endure? What would I do with my time? These are the tough questions we often ask ourselves as we approach the end of work we've loved and that has defined us in many ways. But the truth was that for the most part, I'd already answered them following my unchosen departure from my job.

At sixty, my pension from the time I'd worked in the federal government in the 1970s and '80s kicked in. Though modest, I crunched the numbers and figured out that if I combined it with my reduced CLC pension, I'd have an adequate income.

My decision to retire (I prefer the Spanish *jubilado*) this summer was a convergence of many things from the practical to the spiritual. In the end, it was about "carpe diem," about seizing the moment, following my heart, and making every day count, whether I have two more years to live or twenty. I don't necessarily see it as the end of work per se, but the end of working full-time and the beginning of a vibrant new chapter.

An offshoot of my original breast cancer support group continues to meet once a month or so for breakfast. It remains a rich source of support and information, and because of our shared experience, a place where we can laugh one moment and weep the next. It's a gathering of the Breast Friends, as we now call ourselves, like none other.

I planted a small garden this spring. I had hoped to plant a vegetable garden last year, and dug up a plot in the backyard and got it ready for planting. Then I crashed, and there was no garden. My garden, like getting my portocath out, is symbolic of new beginnings and possibilities, a planting of seeds and seedlings. May some of them grow and flourish this time.

It's time to say *au revoir* for now. Please know how important you've been and continue to be in my healing and my life.

Be well. Carpe diem.
Love, Tamara

Reflections

CELEBRATING RETIREMENT

Once I'd finally made up my mind to retire, I called to tell my director right away. We got together for coffee shortly thereafter, and it was a lovely surprise when he said he wanted to organize a party in my honor, as we had never worked together directly and I'd been gone from work for almost two years. I was moved by his thoughtfulness and pleased at the idea of having some kind of ritual to mark this transition. It occurred to me that it would also be a way for me to leave when I was feeling well and unbroken. When he asked what kind of party I wanted, my only request was that it be warm and low-key and that it include friends and colleagues from various parts of my life. Ideally, it would take place in the CLC building so my co-workers could stop by on their way home from work.

A team of my friends at the CLC and from other unions got together to plan it, and when I walked into the board room on the day of the party, I could hardly believe my eyes. The board room tables were no longer arranged in the usual hollow square, but were set up café-style, with bright tablecloths, flowers, and candles. A table was laden with a spread of tantalizing appetizers and drinks. Samples of my work from the previous fifteen years were everywhere: literacy newsletters, films, posters, and publications were on display. A beautiful mobile made of colorful literacy bookmarks hung from the ceiling. Best of all, Larry, Rachel, co-workers, and friends had gathered from work and other parts of my life.

Barb, the CLC Vice-President with whom I'd worked closely in literacy and education, was the emcee. She welcomed everyone and then followed with a glowing tribute. Cathy facilitated a word café session, where people were invited to gather around the café tables to discuss questions like "What inspires you about Tamara?" After they'd written down what they had come up with on small pieces of paper, Cathy invited them to share with the group what they'd discussed or written down. Then she collected the papers into a beautiful wooden box and gave it to me. Elaine, my secretary, read aloud excerpts from poems and songs I'd written over the years, and for each one I had to guess the person I'd written it for. Bev facilitated a session where everyone called out their associations with the letters of my name. A friend brought his guitar and got everyone to sing along with some favorite songs.

Later, a group gathered at Barb's house for a fabulous supper, spilling out on to her patio into the balmy summer night. After we'd eaten, I invited everyone to come and sit in a circle in the living room. I went around the circle, recounting a story about my connection with each person there. Completely spontaneously, after I'd told a story about someone, each of them responded in turn with an anecdote or memory of their own. By the time we reached the end of the circle, each of us felt connected to everyone else there. It was well past midnight when we finally said good night, and I was already over the moon.

Through my cancer experience, I have come to know and appreciate who I am apart from my job. I revel in exploring and deepening my multiple roles as mother, wife, daughter, sister, friend, confidante, caregiver, writer, advocate, learner, facilitator, activist, reader, correspondent, board member, music lover, walker, cyclist, swimmer, songstress, novice gardener, nature lover, cook, traveler, Upwords player, etc. I've learned that for the most part, the relationships that really matter have endured, and most of those that have fallen by the wayside probably weren't that important anyway. I've discovered that filling my time isn't a problem as there is so much I want to do, and instead, my challenge is how to focus on what makes my heart sing the most.

I'm also realizing how important rituals were to me throughout my cancer journey. When there wasn't a ready-made ritual available, we'd try to figure one out that fit the rite of passage for which it was required. There were many rituals along the way: my sister's arrival for my post-chemo weekends, the shiva and memorial after my dad's death, the healing circle, ringing the chemo bell, hosting the thank you party, and celebrating my retirement, and writing my Healing Journey letters. Singing was an integral part of most of them. Playing Upwords and writing the letters became rituals. Each marked an occasion, a transition, or a turning point and gave it deeper meaning.

ROLE REVERSALS

While I steadily gained strength, it was alarming to watch Larry's health deteriorating at the same time. The pain in his thighs he'd been dealing with for years had become worse and was debilitating at times. Based on a couple of MRI results, his pain had been attributed to spinal stenosis putting pressure on his sciatic nerve. He finally saw an orthopedic surgeon, expecting to be heading for back surgery to resolve the problem. But after a thorough examination, the surgeon was unconvinced that the major problem was orthopedic, and referred Larry to a vascular specialist.

A few weeks later, the vascular surgeon diagnosed Peripheral Arterial Disease (PAD), a hardening of the arteries that had reduced the circulation in his legs and pelvis to only 50 percent. The verdict was unequivocal: Larry would have to quit smoking immediately, and he would need an angioplasty and possibly bypass surgery to deal with the blockages in both of his legs. He quit smoking the next day. He had the vascular surgery but has since been diagnosed with severe arthritis in both hips, necessitating replacement surgery.

Almost overnight, our roles reversed. Just two years before, we had been independent, healthy adults. Then I became a cancer patient with Larry as my primary caregiver. Now that Larry was dealing with his own health problems, I had to cross the bridge from patient to caregiver. The only good thing about it was that we hadn't both been ill at the same time.

I noticed how Larry was handling his health crisis differently this time. When he'd had complications from an enlarged prostate the year before, he'd retreated to deal with the pain on his own. He hadn't wanted to talk about what was happening to him and didn't want me to go with him to his appointments with the urologist. But this time, he asked me to go to all his medical appointments. We discussed strategies and options, getting together beforehand to work out questions to take to his doctors.

I was glad to be there for Larry and to be developing a new kind of partnership around our health. Armed with a growing knowledge of how the health care system works and about how to become captains of our own ships, "in sickness and in health" was taking on new meaning for both of us.

It was also devastating to get the news of my friend Debbie's endometrial cancer. She had been such a constant support to me when I was sick and in treatment the year before, and now she too was facing a cancer diagnosis, a hysterectomy and radiation treatment. After her surgery and before radiation started, Deb wondered whether it wouldn't be simpler to drive herself to her daily appointments, at least at the beginning.

Speaking from experience, I encouraged her to accept the rides from friends because it would be a chance for her to have short visits, even if she didn't need them in the practical sense. When Deb agreed to try it out, Denise organized a meal schedule and I put the rides together. It was good for me to take the driver's seat again. With friends volunteering, Deb felt loved and supported throughout one of the toughest times in her life. I was gratified when Judy said we had all learned about how to create a support system because of me.

It was a strange reversal of roles to become the caregiver so soon after being the patient. Was it a coincidence, or was it that our age group was suddenly hitting the wall with major health issues? I was glad to be well enough to help out wherever I could.

IN GRATITUDE: RUNNING FOR THE CURE

As time went on, I realized there were many ways to express my gratitude for my current healthy status and for all that had been done for me. I was delighted when Linda, the social worker at the Women's Breast Health Centre, invited me to come as a resource person to a breast cancer support group for newly diagnosed women. It was a gratifying experience for me. The women were sitting on the same comfortable floral-patterned couches arranged in a circle in the hospital lounge where my own support group had gathered a year and half before. Conscious of the full head of hair I now had, I wondered what it would be like for the women there who were wearing wigs, bandanas, and woolly hats. But I think my hair gave them hope. From the moment I sat down to join them, we were sisters.

I only had half an hour to spend with them, so I'd decided to read a few bits from my Healing Journey letters out loud. After each piece, I invited them to share their thoughts and experiences on a theme that had emerged, like losing our hair, the chemo paradox, finding strength in vulnerability. I also picked up on one of Joyce's questions, asking, "What nourishes you during this time?" and told the group about how writing my letters through my treatment had been an important part of my healing.

The enthusiastic response to the session and others I went to in the months that followed made me realize that there could be multiple uses for my letters. I mused about what it might be like to lead a writing group for breast cancer patients and wondered about other roles I might play within the cancer healing community.

Over the years, I'd sponsored friends who had walked and run to raise money to fight breast cancer, and I had been moved when some had walked or run in my name. Last year, I'd been in Greece at the time of the annual Run for the Cure, but now I was feeling well and wanted to help raise funds. I also wanted to experience the visceral solidarity of being in a groundswell of support for women who were experiencing or had gone through breast cancer. This included those who were no longer with us, and I was determined to walk in honor of Martha.

A request to friends and family raised almost $1,200 in less than a week. It felt good that I'd be walking with MARTHA printed in bold letters on the sign I'd be wearing on a string around my neck on the day of the run.

The early October morning of the run was gray, drizzly, and cold, so I put on long underwear and stuffed a yellow rain poncho into my knapsack along with a water bottle and camera. I had coffee and muffins ready at our house at 7:30 in the morning for my friends who would be joining me. When we arrived at Lebreton Flats, I was astonished to see the size of the crowd and how it was awash in shocking pink, the brightly colored feathers, hats, and costumes vibrant against the gray sky. There were thousands of people of all ages, from young kids to grandparents, in strollers and wheelchairs and on foot, milling about, checking out the freebies at the sponsors' tables, horsing around, chatting, and laughing.

I'd registered for the run as a survivor, so I'd received an invitation to come early for a photo shoot at the "Survivors' Wall" before the run was to start. I walked over to it alone, approaching it gingerly. Dozens of women's names were written all over it, and I stood there reading them in silence, thinking about Martha. Survivors were starting to congregate, so I joined them in one of the back rows for the photo.

When the woman standing beside me asked me when I'd been diagnosed, I told her it had been in the summer of 2009. She introduced herself, saying she was from Saskatchewan and that she'd been diagnosed in 1993. "Wow," I said, "and you're here!"

"Yes, and I'm well," she answered, as an exuberant smile lit up her face, "Here with my daughter and granddaughter." Tears flowed as we embraced and I thought of Martha, the woman from Saskatchewan, and me – and the cruel game of roulette that decides each of our fates.

Before the day of the run, I had been in touch with Laurie Kingston, a breast cancer survivor. I'd been moved by her book *Not Done Yet* about her cancer experience when I'd read it the year before. We found Laurie and the members of her team sporting T-shirts emblazoned with their team name *No pink for profit*.

There had been a spread in the *Ottawa Citizen* the day before about the team and what it stood for. The article talked about how Laurie and some of her friends had felt "exploited by the big pink merchandising machine" and had decided to do something about it. Angry about the deluge of pink, they started thinking about the politics of a color that has become shorthand for the "tyranny of passive consumerism."

Laurie told me that when she was diagnosed in 2006 at age thirty-eight, she was thrust into the politicized world of cancer. Inundated by well-meaning friends who gave her pink trinkets, she couldn't help feeling that cancer had become an opportunity to sell pink products, of which only a tiny percentage of the profit goes to research. "It's a cynical way for these corporations to raise their own profile," she said.

Even worse are the companies that engage in "pinkwashing." Another survivor on Laurie's team said she'd rather people make a conscious decision to stop putting pesticides on their lawn. "It's a small thing," she said. "Forget the pink ribbon. Don't put poison on your property."

Laurie still wanted to be part of the Run for the Cure. "It's a fun event. But we're uncomfortable with some of the pink stuff that's everywhere during Breast Cancer Awareness month." I thought she had come up with a brilliant solution that addressed her concerns while still participating in the run by creatively naming the team 'No pink for profit' and getting the word out. As Laurie said, "We hate the pink machine, but we hate breast cancer more."

It was 9 a.m., time for the run to start. The skies had cleared a bit, and a few rays of sun were starting to poke through. With my trusty crew, we headed for the start of the route for the five-kilometer walk. My head was spinning with everything that was happening – the solidarity, the spirit, the contradictions, the memories of Martha. We linked arms, smiled broadly, and forged ahead.

IMAGINING A BETTER SYSTEM

Finding the lump in my underarm, then another lump in my breast, and thinking I might have breast cancer was horrible enough. But waiting in dread for weeks for a diagnosis and then for several more weeks trying to get on the right track for treatment was an excruciating time. These pre- and post-diagnosis times were not only wrought with anxiety. As I creaked open the door to the world of breast cancer, it would be here that I'd encounter the longest wait times and the most convoluted processes throughout my journey with cancer.

In the letter I wrote to the Women's Breast Health Centre a few weeks after my diagnosis, I described some of the difficulties I had experienced over the previous three months. I put forward the idea of the nurse navigator. "Could the Centre assign each new patient to a nurse navigator from the time of her diagnosis so that someone is there to advocate on her behalf at one of the most stressful times in her life?" I asked: "If I was so utterly lost at such a critical time, what was happening to the women who had little confidence, support, or education? What if they didn't speak English?" Along with my suggestions, I wanted my letter to convey how much I believed in the Centre: "My fervent hope is that my observations prove to be helpful in your efforts to provide optimal health care and support to women like me."

> **Dr. Shailendra Verma:** What we tend to do now is to send you to the social worker to have your cry. But what we've found is that the best way to deal with anxiety is not handholding but knowledge. Women are incredibly strong. As long as they know what's happening and what they need to do, they can organize their families, their jobs, and their lives and get on with it.

> **Dr. Joanne Meng:** We need communication across the historic silos in the hospital system.

When I talked to other women about their experiences, often their particular paths had been somewhat different from mine, with most having surgery before chemotherapy. But almost every one of us seems to have experienced some version of the "black hole" from the outset of our pre- and post-diagnostic processes. The fear and uncertainty continued until our treatment plan was put in place.

There are financial and many other issues involved in looking at any aspect of the health care system. But I don't think money is the primary source of the problem. Rather, the main issue seems to be a lack of co-ordination both among the various specialists and the silos – those separate departments with their own staff and ways of doing things – operating within the hospital. In addition, complementary medicine remains separate from hospital treatment and care and lacks the support of public health care dollars. But let's dream for a moment. If we were to imagine a better process for even just these critical pre-treatment steps, what would it look like?

In the dream, there is a center where women go for "one-stop shopping" for all the diagnostic and planning steps leading up to treating their breast cancer. We would go there as soon as we have inkling there might be a problem, a suspicious lump, an abnormal mammogram result, breast pain, etc. It is also a place to go if we are high-risk patients. Our family doctor has briefed us about thoroughly about what lies ahead and has referred us to the center.

Ideally, we are accompanied to the center by a family member

> **Dr. Joanne Meng:** Family doctors should be able to counsel their patients about the process of navigating the initial stages of the cancer care system and explain what they might entail. They should be able to advise their patients about the tests they will go through, why and what the wait times will be. There needs to be better rapport between family doctors and cancer specialists. Sometimes family doctors feel like we only call them when the patient is dying and we want them to relay the bad news.

or friend. We are warmly greeted by a nurse who has been specially trained for her role as "navigator" and who has taken the time to become thoroughly familiar with our file. She examines us, bringing in a doctor as required. Afterward, she advises us of what lies ahead, at least in the short term, and arranges for diagnostic tests. She is available to us throughout the journey, giving us her contact information so we can call or consult her at any step along the way.

> **Dr. Angel Arnaout:** Our hope is to have a nurse for every patient.

All manner of diagnostic tools and equipment are available at the center, along with the medical and technical staff to carry out the required mammograms, ultrasounds, CT scans, MRIs, biopsies, etc. Radiologists and other specialists are available to read the scans so the patient can quickly move on to the next step as required. There is ready access to a laboratory where our biopsies can be examined by pathologists and the results determined. The results and/or the diagnosis, available within a day or two, are communicated to us in person within the next couple of days by the nurse navigator. If we have breast cancer, she explains what it might mean in terms of treatment.

> **Dr. Angel Arnaout:** The first goal is to try to get it all on the same day. If we get it all on the same day, you don't have weeks waiting in between, and we can all assess your response together.

Over the next few days, the specifics of the plan are discussed by a team of specialists at a multi-disciplinary meeting or "round." The specialists include the medical oncologist, the surgeon, the radiation oncologist, and the naturopathic oncologist as well as the nurse navigator and possibly the pathologist, radiologist, and others as required. They consider the test results in light of the medical history of the patient, who is encouraged to be present. As much information as possible is shared about the particular nature of the patient's cancer, and the risks and benefits of each possible direction are discussed, explored, and explained. A decision about a plan and a timeframe for treating the patient is reached, ideally by consensus, and arrangements are made to implement it as soon as possible.

> Dr. Angel Arnaout: There should be some type of system where the loop closes. You would be sitting in a conference room, along with all of us at once, where a plan is discussed all at the same time.

> Dr. Shailendra Verma: Our goal should be to come up with the best treatment plan with the least disfigurement and the least suffering.

After the multidisciplinary round, the nurse navigator meets with us again and answers any questions we might have. She communicates clearly in lay language what is known about our cancer and what the treatment plan will entail. If there is not a single clear direction, the risks and benefits of the various options are explained. She outlines what the treatment will involve, how we might prepare for it, how we will receive it, the side effects that might occur, which drugs are available to deal with the side effects, etc. She also offers us information and resources about counseling services, support groups, exercise, yoga, meditation, naturopathic oncology, and other complementary therapies. The nurse navigator continues to be available to us as needed, checking in with us regularly as our treatment progresses.

As patients, we are empowered by the health care system to ensure we get the best care possible. Our treatment is planned to target our individual set of conditions. Throughout our journey, we are considered as whole persons, as women being treated for a disease that is wreaking havoc in every aspect of our beings. Our physical, psychological, emotional, and sexual health is the primary focus of all decisions regarding how our care is compassionately planned and delivered.

Once we are through treatment, there is sufficient recovery time and other supports in place to help us rebuild our health and our lives as we reintegrate into the workplace and community. We will do this in a way that maintains and fosters our health.

> Dr. Shailendra Verma: If we put the effort in at the front end, it will pay off at the other end.

AN IMPROVED REALITY

While there is still a long way to go, some positive changes are starting to happen. At the Women's Breast Health Centre, for example, all cases of locally advanced breast cancer now go to multi-disciplinary rounds as a matter of course. Most of these patients are starting their treatment with chemotherapy.

> Dr. Shailendra Verma: There have been some dramatic changes here as well as globally. The way we look at breast cancer has changed. There's less territoriality. In the case of locally advanced breast cancers, we now try to figure out how we can harness the disease before we harness the breast.

Also at the Ottawa Hospital, a pilot project is underway to bring in the role of the nurse navigator for colorectal cancer patients. The hope is to learn from the pilot and that the navigational model will become more widespread within the hospital and beyond. As we learn more about the complexity of breast cancer, a trend is growing toward approaching each patient as "one woman, one cancer, one treatment." The goal is to look at the situation of each patient and to develop an individualized treatment plan.

Dr. Shailendra Verma: It means a major shift in organizational processes. When you take a biopsy, it's not enough to say, "It's breast cancer." It means finding the hospital resources to allocate the time of the pathologists to do the extra lab work to analyze the biopsy results to determine the markers of each woman's cancer. Then you have to find the pathway that makes it meaningful because once you have identified the problem, you have to find a solution.

In my community, the Maplesoft Centre is a vibrant new cancer survivorship center has opened recently with a vast array of excellent non-medical programs free of charge. In addition to support groups and exercise and nutrition programs, it has cancer coaches on staff who are available to help patients navigate their way through the system. At the same time, the Ottawa Integrative Cancer Centre (OICC) is an exciting holistic integrative cancer center that has recently opened its doors to offer a wide range of complementary cancer care. This includes oncological naturopathy, physiotherapy, massage therapy, acupuncture, and family therapy as well as courses in nutrition, meditation, and yoga. A project of the Canadian College of Naturopathic Medicine, it is carrying out research, training oncological naturopaths, and building bridges to mainstream oncology. Dr. Leesa Kirchner is Chief Clinical Medical Officer there along with two of my other doctors who are actively involved in the OICC. Dr. Shailendra Verma is a member of the OICC's Scientific Advisory Board and Dr. Angel Arnaout is a principal investigator in a study on the role of vitamin D in preventing and fighting cancer.

I feel hopeful about these positive developments. There is growing interest in preventing cancer, in developing ways to support the body's inherent ability to heal, and in addressing the needs of the whole person. Efforts are underway to foster multidisciplinary approaches to treatment and to promote wellness. Breast cancer patients and survivors are advocating for prevention, better treatment and support, and complementary care.

While I can't know what the future will bring, I'm feeling hopeful about it. Whatever hills, valleys, and plateaus may lie ahead, I'll be carrying the spirit of *carpe diem* with me as I look forward to seizing the wonder of each new day of my life.

Be well. Carpe diem.
Love, Tamara

Voices of the Healers

Three amazing doctors and a naturopath worked with me throughout my illness and thereafter. Over time, I developed a relationship with each of them. During my "year from hell" they examined me and wanted to know how I was dealing with cancer and responding to treatment. Sometimes, they asked me about what was going on in my life. I also worked with a life coach who played a different but equally significant part in my healing journey.

Afterward, I was interested in finding out what it was like from their vantage point. Why do they do this work? How do they see breast cancer? What about their relationships with their patients? How do they cope with losing some of them? I asked about their views on integrating mainstream and complementary medicine and about what keeps them going in the face of loss. I also interviewed my life coach about how she supports her clients who are going through breast cancer. I was curious about what they believe is working in the system of cancer care and what needs to change.

Once my recovery period was over and I was starting to write *But Hope is Longer*, I asked these members of my "team" if they would meet with me. I was thrilled when they each agreed to give me some of their precious time.

DR. SHAILENDRA VERMA, MEDICAL ONCOLOGIST

I will always be grateful to Dr. Verma for putting me on the treatment path that was best for me. He was in charge of planning my chemotherapy, monitoring my progress, and co-ordinating my overall treatment. A brilliant doctor and compassionate human being, he continues to monitor me with regular follow-up appointments three years after my diagnosis.

Dr. Shailendra Verma graduated from Queen's University as an MD in 1979. In 1985, after post-graduate training in internal medicine, hematology, and oncology, he began to practice at the Ottawa Hospital Cancer Centre and became an associate professor at the Faculty of Medicine, University of Ottawa. Since then, Dr. Verma has held many regional, provincial, and national responsibilities and posts. These include playing an active role in the Canadian Breast Cancer Foundation and the Scientific Advisory Board of the Ottawa Integrative Cancer Centre. A committed advocate on behalf of breast cancer patients in policy, research, and treatment, he values above all the delivery of timely, evidence-based, and compassionate care of his patients from whom he continues to gather inspiration and insight.

> **Dr. Verma:** When I started in oncology almost thirty years ago, it was a new specialty. Little was known, and I was drawn to it because it was on the cusp of discovery. It also spoke to me of a certain tenderness. I never had children, so it gave me the maternal and paternal flavors that I enjoy in medicine. I felt this was my niche. Everyone I worked with at the time, whether I

was a medical student, an intern, or a resident, always seemed to comment on the compassion that I brought into medicine. So I always felt that this was the right place for me to be, a place where there was a need for discovery and a need for care. What better place than oncology?

In the beginning, I did everything: breast cancer, leukemia, lymphoma, melanoma, and sarcoma of young patients. Breast cancer, by virtue of its volume, became my bread and butter, so to speak. I was particularly drawn to breast cancer. Before we recognized that it was not one but many illnesses because of the different types of breast cancer, I always described how the face of breast cancer was different in every clinic I went to. I might see a young woman, an older woman, a mother, a widow, a lesbian, a teenager: it drew me because it was already a different disease for each woman. It became a very intimate illness for me.

I advocated from the very beginning for any advance that might help in breast cancer. I played a role in every possible aspect of breast cancer: in genetics, research, prevention, screening, pathology, markers, etc. I believe as doctors, we have to be advocates for our patients, for everything from how money should be spent to how care should be delivered. If you're really passionate about it, you delve into every part of this disease so that the patient in 2020 gets even better care than in 2012 because of what you've done.

Losing a patient is never easy. You grieve for them, you grieve with them, you love them. But you maintain the strength. You keep reiterating in your own mind "Could I have done something different? Was something overlooked?" But at this time when nothing more can be done, I find that what helps me the most is to witness myself not as hero, but as rock, the person that people can depend on. I don't want to rush in there and save the life anymore, because I can't. I've never seen myself as, "I can rush in and give you the magic serum."

There are times that you feel real pain. I don't want my patients to develop metastatic disease. What helps me weather this is a sense of commiseration – a real bonding with them and reassuring them that I will do my best to come up with the next step in the plan. And if I can't, I will get the right person who can. I don't think anyone in the world can say, "Well I know everything about heart disease and I'll stop you from having a heart attack." It's the same for an oncologist.

A lot of people express a lot of care for their caregivers. It's a tender moment for me. I never lose sight of the fact that I don't walk into a room asking for a patient to be sad for me. That's too much of a role reversal. On the other hand, it's a remarkable progress of humankind that patient and physician can sit and talk to each other as two human beings, that there isn't this separation of church and state so to speak. I think we need to respect the fact that many of our patients are sophisticated in their thinking, that they're knowledgeable and have a mastery of so many things that we don't have as physicians.

What physicians have is the ability to open a few doors. I can open the door to surgery. I can write a prescription for chemotherapy. These are not lax powers, and we respect that. But at the end of the day, we have to respect the fact that those are simply abilities. Knowledge, on the other hand, is something that transcends all of that. I've come to respect that enormously.

I think we should be able to teach this, and I think it comes from recognizing two things. One: There's no difference between the doctor and the patient. We are the same. There's an artificial divide that's been created, and people call that empathy, but it's much more than that. Two: I, the physician, don't know everything. If you enter the room with a bit of humility, there's a huge calm that enters with you.

I had a high-school sports injury with my front tooth. When my dentist was finally taking out the tooth thirty-five years later, he said, "I don't know how you do what you do as an oncologist." I said, "You're pulling my tooth out, and you're telling me you don't know how I do it. Listen, there's a lot of joy in my work, a huge amount of joy."

DR. LEESA KIRCHNER, NATUROPATHIC ONCOLOGIST

From the time I met Dr. Kirchner, I knew I wanted to work with her. She had years of training and experience working with cancer patients despite being in her mid-thirties, and she was one of only a handful of certified naturopathic oncologists in Canada. I was convinced that the skills and therapies she had to offer would serve me well both in fighting my cancer and in diminishing the side effects of treatment. I also believed that her support would complement the medical care I'd be getting through the cancer center. Combined with healthy food and exercise, I would be doing what I could to get well. She invited me to call her Leesa.

Leesa was drawn to working with cancer patients because she believes naturopathic medicine has something important to offer in addition to conventional medicine. She gives hope but never false hope, and values the strong relationships she develops with her patients. She came to tears when she talked about the losses among her patients that are almost unbearable. One of the ways she copes is to take frequent holidays. Leesa also has a wonderfully dry sense of humor that helps get all of us through the rough times.

Dr. Leesa Kirchner graduated as a naturopathic doctor in 2003 from the Canadian College of Naturopathic Medicine in Toronto. She was awarded the status of Fellow of the American Board of Naturopathic Oncology (FABNO). Leesa ran a successful general family practice before deciding to focus her work exclusively on naturopathic oncology in 2006, a role she finds both challenging and rewarding. In Alberta, Leesa completed post-graduate training in intravenous therapies for the treatment of cancer and is currently involved in a research project to further explore the role of IV vitamin C in patients with cancer. As the chief clinical medical officer at the Ottawa Integrative Cancer Centre (OICC), Leesa is keen to advance whole-person cancer care and believes strongly in the ability of the OICC to help affect real change.

Leesa: I don't think I saw a single cancer patient during my internship or residency. When I started working in Alberta after I graduated, they were running an IV clinic. A cancer patient came through the door and said "I really want to try intravenous vitamin C." Nobody knew much about it, so we looked into it and realized it had promise.

When I moved to Ontario and started a general practice, I had a thirty-year-old patient with Stage IV malignant melanoma who was told there was nothing more they could do. By then, I knew quite a bit about the benefits of vitamin C. As we were doing the drips, we had really in-depth discussions. We got to know each other and enjoyed our time together. He became a friend. A few years later, he went back to work and his wife got pregnant. He got to have quite a few good years after cancer, but he ended up with brain metastasis a few years later and died, which was horrible.

During that time, I realized that as much as working with cancer was difficult, I found I had a hard time sympathizing to the same extent with the people who came in with minor problems. If someone said, "I have to lose ten pounds," I'd want to say, "Well, go run or something." I found myself thinking, "You're not dying, so get over it." The connections I had with cancer patients were different. They were powerful. I decided

I wanted to work exclusively with cancer patients even though every part of my brain was saying, "Why are you picking the hardest thing on earth?" But I didn't pick it, it picked me.

It's tough when my patients want integrative treatment and their oncologists are negative about it. It scares them when they don't have the approval of their oncologist, so they end up in an internal battle. They come to see me and say, "I trust you and I know what you're saying. But I'm scared, and I don't know what to do." I don't know if there's a single answer because everyone is different. Some people raise the possibility of complementary care with their doctors and then get shot down. Then they say "Forget it, I'm not telling you anything anymore." Others say "I'm not doing anything unless I have a 100 percent seal of approval from my oncologist." So it's where people fit on the continuum and how they deal with it.

In the five years since I've been focusing on oncology, I've seen a huge shift. Not only in oncologists' attitudes, but also in patient education. Patients know naturopathic support is available, that it will help them, and they're determined to get it. Oncologists know it's happening. The bottom line is that people are doing it.

I had a patient yesterday tell me her doctor had never seen anyone tolerate as many rounds of chemo as she had in her situation. It was beyond anything she should have been able to do. It's because she's using so many complementary strategies to support her that she's able to do that. I had another patient recently who was working with me prior to having a bone marrow transplant. Her oncologist had been very open and said, "You should see a naturopath because you need to work on your immune system, and I don't know how." When they started neuro-harvesting her cells, she had three times more cells than they had ever retrieved from anyone before. She was supposed to be in the hospital for two weeks. When she came out in two days, they said, "This is nine days quicker than our record."

A lot of the shift comes from stories like these because the oncologists are seeing it for themselves. People are using complementary care, then they're going to see their oncologists. The oncologists are seeing the difference for themselves.

I hope that in the future, our focus will shift from not only killing cancer cells, but also to supporting the body more completely throughout the process. It will be about managing side effects without causing others with the treatment, teaching patients the importance of exercise and diet, and keeping patients healthy both physically and emotionally through the process. And, hopefully, it will empower patients so that when treatment is over they are not simply waiting for the next CT scan to tell them if the cancer is back. It will give them tools to actively lower the risk of recurrence so they can move on with their lives feeling that they are being proactive. My hope is that this becomes the norm in cancer care. I don't want my role to be completely eliminated, but I would like these basic things to be available to all patients, not just those who seek it out.

JOYCE HARDMAN, LIFE COACH

I went back to see Joyce Hardman, life coach, in 2008. It had been seven years since I'd first worked with her and a year before I was diagnosed. I highly valued her role in my life as a wise guide and mentor as well as a powerful coach. When I learned I had cancer, I knew Joyce would have a great deal to offer me now, especially since she had accompanied several other breast cancer patients on their journeys.

Joyce Hardman has been in full-time practice as a life coach since

1998. She has a master's degree in education along with extensive training and certification in coaching. From her years of being a workshop leader and holistic counselor, she brings wisdom and facilitation skills that include deep listening and the ability to understand and articulate the stages and challenges of human transformation.

Joyce: Coaching is about helping people discover what their vision of happiness is and supporting them as they move in that direction. It's about choosing one's destiny more carefully and soulfully and moving toward it. It also has a spiritual component, because the most powerful way to move toward one's destiny is to be in balance with the whole, to be in a relationship with all of life.

In some situations, the route to happiness is at a basic level, and that will be the starting place of coaching. For example, someone wants to find a partner or a new job or a specific condition of happiness. They're clarifying their dream, learning the skills of moving toward it. They're finding out more about themselves as they notice what they might be doing that is getting in the way and learning how to deal with it. Slowly, they begin to get the spiritual part. But when they get a diagnosis of breast cancer, they are preoccupied with getting healthy and staying alive. They focus on what's happening now rather than on some future scenario. The question isn't "How do I get somewhere down the road in my life?" but rather "What does it take to be whole?"

I remember telling you at the beginning that every woman I've watched go through this, even though she hated the cancer, has come away saying, "I've changed in a way I never would have changed before." We put that on hold in the beginning because the first and necessary stage in this walk is to be angry and frustrated. What's happening isn't fair or just. There's a sense that there is no caring underpinning to life. It's a killer of faith in the beginning, because we believe in the certainties we take for granted. We make assumptions about our certainties like, "I'm taking care of my body, so I won't get sick." Then we find out we have cancer, and who knows what's certain anymore? We put our faith in these certainties, and they crash. But the crashing is actually a gateway.

On the practical side, there's the question of balance, of discovering what's out of balance for us, what makes balance. In a way, people with cancer have been separated from their lives. At a time when you want to create more balance so your healing will go well, we can look and ask "Where is the balance off here?" Each person has different ways that their balance is off. Your way has always been around your need for spaciousness. For you, it's the play between finding spaciousness and helping to change the world and connecting with people. You've been working with that tension all the way through and discovering lots of new territory.

The answer has a lot to do with self-love and self-care. It's about moving away from living out of balance and harmony and diffusing our deep sense of guilt. As we move toward better balance and self-care, somehow everything seems to work better. We're not fighting life so much.

Sometimes life brings us to a place where we decide to walk into something painful, like chemo. We have to leave an abusive husband or a toxic workplace, we have to do something in order to survive or for some greater purpose. And then that pain changes from the devil to an angel. It's your angel because it is the absolute thing you must be doing. If chemo is the best treatment available right now, it's what you have to do to sustain your life. So it's your angel, even though many parts of you are screaming "No!" because there is a bigger "Yes."

The "yes" to it, the embrace of it, the trust that it is taking you where you are supposed to be going in your transformation, in your evolution, and even in your healing actually makes it so. Your body then goes "yes" as opposed to "no."

There is such an allergy to rest that's there for everyone, especially for women. I find women feeling guilty about not going back to work, guilty about not helping out more. Even if it's not guilt, it's about how hard it is to rest, to pause, to stop. Then there's the discovery, once you do rest, of how that very simple thing is so powerful. It's not something to be afraid of, it's not a waste of time. It's like really good soil.

Most women who get the diagnosis want to keep on doing everything possible in the physical, emotional, and spiritual realms. They feel compelled to carry on with all that they do because women are the nurturers and caretakers. After chemo, they think they're supposed to be washing the carpets because that's what they do every May. But they forget how important it is to say "I can only do what I can do. I also need to rest."

I'm there to remind them that this is a special year. It's as if you're on a pilgrimage like the Camino. You don't clean your carpets while you're walking the Camino.

The question "What is cancer all about?" makes me ponder. Following a garden metaphor, it is an unimpeded overgrowth. It's like a plant pushing out tons of flowers when the conditions are not good in the air or soil because it wants to preserve itself by creating lots of seeds. But at the same time, it also depletes itself because the seed growth is at the expense of the leaves and stems. So the call is for a healthier environment in which to nourish the whole plant.

My hope is that cancer in the near future will be seen as a signal that the environment is lacking the right nourishment. First, we need to find ways to nourish the one who is "the canary," the

But Hope is Longer

cancer patient who is bearing the overgrowth. Second, I hope we will wake up as a society and look at what is missing. In a male-dominated world, what nourishes is often disregarded, resulting, for example, in the undervaluing of jobs that care for and educate our children. It is expressed in the devaluing of the environment and the lack of ability to relate with other humans.

My hope is that we will find ways that cease to punish cancer patients with poison chemicals and rays, which make them the sacrificial lambs for society's unconscious focus on consumption rather than on co-creating a good life. Attacking the cancer and the patient gives the illusion that we are doing something. Instead, the real solution lies in building societal and environmental health.

I want to express my appreciation of you, who you were when you walked through this, and your receptivity. I was astounded walking through it with you. Life was so thunderous. Some people get their transformational opportunities all along, like if they have really crappy childhoods. But you seemed to get this quadruple whammy all at once. You had a lot of good conditions with friends and sisters along with the challenges. Things were fairly stable and you had a good healthy strong body. And then wham!

It was amazing for me to walk next to you through your transformational pilgrimage. It was like the Camino, only harder. Way harder because you didn't know if you were going to make it at times. The honesty in which you walked it: you weren't mad just once, you were going to be mad a lot and you had to keep on letting go. The realization that it wasn't a permanent fix, that you just had to keep doing it and claim space and boundaries, again and again. You had to simplify, simplify, simplify, and it kept going and going. It was a pounding learning for you. I respected how you did it, how you were willing to keep going. Sometimes it was as minimal as "Well I guess I'm still alive, so I'll keep on going today."

I think you even prepared yourself to be able to write this book, to book off time to do something so internal. To take the ego-burn of being edited and having impossible deadlines. We were coaching about this stuff years ago to be able to have boundaries so you could go and do inner work. And now you're doing it.

DR. ANGEL ARNAOUT, BREAST CANCER SURGEON

At my first appointment with Dr. Arnaout at the Women's Breast Health Centre, I was immediately struck by her beauty. I guessed she was in her late thirties, with clear olive skin and dark eyes. After she examined me thoroughly, Karen and I sat around a table with her in an adjoining room. The "Angel," as I would come to call her, offered the option of doing a lumpectomy rather than a mastectomy. She said it would yield similar results. While she confirmed that my cancer was triple negative, she also assured me that I had good reason to be hopeful, and that I was in good hands. After firing the first surgeon I had met with, I was grateful to have an angel looking out for me.

Dr. Angel Arnaout is a Breast Surgical Oncologist at the Ottawa Hospital, Assistant Professor at the University of Ottawa and an Associate Scientist at the Ottawa Hospital Research Institute. She attended Medical School at Dalhousie University and also obtained her General Surgery training in Halifax. She went on to pursue a Masters of Science degree in the Clinician Investigator/Surgeon Scientist Program at the University of Toronto with a Breast Surgical Oncology Fellowship at Sunnybrook Hospital and the Toronto Sunnybrook Regional Cancer Centre. Her clinical interests include improving the quality and access to care of breast cancer patients and oncoplastic breast surgical techniques.

Dr. Arnaout: I trained in general surgery. During my third year, I decided to do some research as part of my training. I wasn't thinking about "breast." The breast cancer research lab was the only lab still available so I went there for six months. Then six months turned into a year, a year turned into two, and the next thing I knew, it was what I was going to do for the rest of my life.

Ninety-nine percent of my work is in breast cancer surgery now. I do as much as I can in breast cancer work. My research is all on breast cancer. Breast cancer research is very exciting, one of the fastest growing research areas in medicine. The biology is exciting because it involves a lot of different angles and different types of molecular biology. It's also exciting because of the advances in surgical techniques and the possibility of linking them to the outlook of the patient, to how she sees herself, and her self-esteem. Ultimately, all the things that traditionally were never measured are now starting to be more important. It has been shown that your cancer outcome improves if you feel better about yourself. The field of breast cancer is fascinating because you get the full spectrum of the basic science part, the hands-on surgical clinical part, and the psycho-social part. In the end, everything connects to improve the outcome for the patient.

We've moved past the old-fashioned way of doing things when a patient would come in saying, "As long as you get rid of the cancer, I don't care how I look or what consequences I have to suffer, as long as I live longer." We know this isn't the whole truth, it's only part of it. Ideally, the whole team is there at the outset, especially with patients whose cancers are locally advanced like yours. It's important for the surgeon to see the patient before she starts treatment. This gives us a sense of the before and after, because what we do at the time of surgery will depend on the patient's response to the chemo or hormonal therapy she has before surgery. Then we have the whole picture, and we're able to talk about the possible surgical options we can offer her.

In your case, I used a surgical technique during your lymph node dissection that, in addition to removing the remnants of cancer, preserved your arm-related lymph nodes. The hope with this technique is to help prevent lymphedema and salvage the range of motion in the affected arm. I believe it is important to take risks like that to take advantage of newer worldwide techniques, even though they may not be fully studied. But you have to be in a situation where you're studying them yourself. I've looked at the outcomes and proved to myself that it's not any worse in terms of oncological data. Clinical trials take at least five to ten years to complete, for the results to come through and get widespread attention. You have to be on top of these things, doing your own clinical data and making sure you are strictly monitoring your patients.

The bottom line is we don't want to cause any harm. We don't want to be in a situation where we're trying new things that have not been technically proven on patients and could potentially put you at a disadvantage. So it's a balance between figuring out what you think is so much better for the patient if it works compared to the risk of potentially leaving disease behind.

I fully support complementary cancer care. None of us have all the answers. We certainly are not able to treat 100 percent of our patients effectively. You need something to top up what we do, which is where the naturopathic approach comes in. The only time I am a little cautious is when there are things that may interfere with the effectiveness of our medications or may actually enhance the growth of cancer. Otherwise, I'm all for it.

I'm excited about a new study we're starting with the Ottawa Integrative Cancer Centre. Everyone knows about the benefits of vitamin D. We know that patients who take vitamin D have less cancer, especially breast and colon cancer, and that patients who end up with breast cancer have lower levels of vitamin D compared to patients who don't have breast cancer. By inferring from those data, you would think that vitamin D is helpful for breast cancer. But we've never been able to study how and why it works and what dosages are best. It's like we're starting out to test a new drug. We want to confirm that it actually kills cancer and prevents cancer. They've just done the same study on prostate cancer. They've shown that the tumor actually does shrink at the high doses we're now investigating in our study.

In North America and Europe, we have mass screening programs. In many other countries this isn't the case, so we are picking up more breast cancer here. That may be why the incidence of breast cancer is higher in Caucasian or white women compared to women from third world countries, for example. It's not so much that the incidence is higher because there's a higher chance if you're a white woman, but because we are actually picking up more. The second thing is that non-white women don't present to us as much because along with cultural taboos, denial, etc., they are less likely to be tapped into the medical system. So they often come to us presenting with a delayed advanced disease.

In my reading of international literature, there is a big push to increase awareness, to change the whole culture of people in understanding that this is not something shameful. Because the breasts are a private part of a woman's body, it is not something they want to share with other people in many parts of the world. Often, the physicians are male, so not only does the patient feel shame at what is happening to her body, but she worries about having to go to a male physician. I think that is part of the reason why they are not presenting.

I don't feel that if we were to do mass screening on these

patients that there would still be a higher incidence in white women. I think it used to be like that because there was a higher incidence of hormone replacement therapy in white women. Some of the risk factors that lead to breast cancer include taking hormone replacement therapy, not bearing children at a younger age, taking birth control pills, and fertility treatments, things which are not readily available to women in third world countries. But these days, women know about breast cancer. When there's anything funny going on with hormones and drugs, they're thinking about the risk factors for breast cancer and think twice about starting it.

My main focus in life is to figure out ways to treat breast cancer. But at the same time, not just to treat it from a medical point of view, but to treat it from a whole person perspective. That's what keeps me going twenty-four hours a day: the joy I get when a woman comes through my clinic, happy, cured, and looking better. I don't think there's any other disease where it is so intrinsically obvious that I will have such a big impact in patients' lives.

DR. JOANNE MENG, RADIATION ONCOLOGIST

Dr. Meng regularly sees hundreds of cancer patients. Probably, many are in crisis and not inclined or able to do much beyond getting through one day at a time. I wonder how she keeps herself going with so much pain and loss going on around her. She is the kind of doctor and person who is always looking for ideas and strategies, medical and otherwise, to support her patients as they travel through diagnosis and treatment. She always took the time to ask me about what else was going on in my life. Dr. Meng is a few years younger than I am. She always calls me Ms. Levine, and of course, I call her

Dr. Meng. After our first few encounters, it seemed strange that she would address me so formally, especially since we were now starting to share something of our lives on a more personal basis. But when I invited her to call me Tamara, she said she didn't feel comfortable doing that as long as I was her patient. Once we had discussed it, we settled amicably into addressing each other by our surnames, at least for now. To myself, I affectionately think of her simply as "Meng."

Dr. Joanne Meng graduated from Memorial University Medical School in 1988. She worked as a General Practitioner in Oncology for many years before pursuing a residency in Radiation Oncology at the University of Ottawa. She became a member of the Ottawa Hospital Cancer Centre in 1999 as well as an Assistant Professor at the University of Ottawa. She is very involved in resident training, and her main interest is to provide the best care she can to her patients.

Dr. Meng: I fell into oncology by accident. I'd worked as a family doctor and didn't really like it. Then a job came up at the cancer clinic as a general practitioner in oncology (GPO). I enjoyed working with colleagues in radiation oncology, and thought, "I can do this, it's interesting work and I think I can help people." I went into it that way, not because I ever set out to be an oncologist.

Cancer patients are not simple patients, they're complex. Whether they're lung cancer or breast cancer patients, there is a complexity because they have cancer. However they respond to it, whether it's "I'm going to die from my lung cancer" or "I'm devastated because I have breast cancer," my job is not a simple "I'm taking your blood pressure because you have hypertension." You can't be just any kind of doctor to do oncology. When there is a diagnosis of cancer, it's automatically perceived as life or death. So you enter into a relationship with the patient that's completely different.

Breast cancer is a highly complex disease, more so than other cancers. With other cancers, like lung cancer, the response from the patient is generally, "Yes, doctor, whatever you say." But with breast cancer, it's catastrophic to women's lives. How does breast cancer impact on a woman's life? How does she reintegrate into her life afterward? Often during treatment, she's in a fog, but afterward she's frantic, which is why some oncologists want to stick to lung cancer. It's so much harder when she feels her sexuality is on the line. She's full of angst, she's weeping, she's put on 40 pounds, her husband is nowhere, her whole world has been turned upside down.

The thing that always strikes me about women with breast cancer is their desire to have the life they had before. They always long for that. They want to know what was wrong with their life before, why they got sick, what they did to bring it on even though they took good care of themselves. There is a lot of self-blame. It's not just breast cancer patients with metastatic disease. Even those women who have a good chance of survival feel the rug was pulled out from under their feet. It's the longing for what was, for their marriage and whatever it might have been. They talk a lot about that when you really ask them.

I don't know if you've ever met anybody with metastatic breast cancer. It's grueling. You're not the same. You don't look the same. You don't feel the same. You've been at the doctor a hundred times. You're on drugs all the time, brutal drugs, and you're on chemo for life. Your husband's worn out. Your family's worn out. Mommy's been sick for as long as your kids can remember.

I have a patient who is forty-one with two young children. She has metastatic breast cancer and it's clipping along at a pretty rapid rate. She recently asked her oncologist what kind of time she has left, and found out she has about a year to live. And that year is going to be a really hard year. It's not that she's going to have a year of her old life and then it's going to be over. It's going to be a hell of a year and it's going to get worse and worse. The prospect of being home when she dies is almost nonexistent.

I said to this woman, "This is really crappy, this is the worst." She's crying, he's crying, I'm crying. That to me is far more devastating than the dying part. I feel terribly sad for these women, not so much about the dying, but about what's happening in relation to her family, her marriage, her work. The dying part is almost a relief sometimes because the suffering is over.

I always worry that in the cases of women with metastatic breast cancer, I'm giving false hope. I'll say we can't get rid of this, but we can control it. I always tell them that our ability to control the disease at this point in medicine is better than it was five or ten years ago. But then I always wonder if I'm giving them some sense of false hope.

I don't always cope with the losses very well. But in oncology, you have to be prepared for failure and loss. We go into medicine expecting we're never going to have failures. We're the high achievers who've never failed. So when you do badly or when people die, you feel it keenly. It's not necessarily that there's something I could personally have done differently or that the system failed, but something failed.

My Vision

My vision has grown out of what I learned in the country of cancer. Cancer is a powerful message in a bottle about the condition of the world we inhabit that raises many questions. What can we learn from a deadly disease that causes normal cells to grow out of control, destroying life-supporting biological processes, and undermining the natural balance of life? What can we do to recreate balance in our own lives and in the life of our planet?

While cancer affects us most directly as individuals and family members, it is fundamentally a social problem. We know enough about cancer to say it has something to do with our relationship to the environment and with how we treat each other. We know the incidence is higher when we live and work in toxic environments: on farms where pesticides are used extensively, in homes and workplaces where asbestos is present, and near waterways polluted by industrial chemicals. We know that greed, excessive consumption, and aggression breed inequality, poverty, hunger, and disease.

In my vision, we each have a role to play as citizens, politicians, policy makers, and health care practitioners in bringing about positive change in our local and global communities. A holistic approach to cancer considers the causes, the treatment options, and the ways to support and rebuild the lives of cancer patients during and after treatment.

Our primary focus is on prevention. Public institutions expose, educate, advocate for, and put regulations in place to that end. When corporations, other institutions, and individuals cause harm to our air, land, and water, they pay a high social price. The consequences are severe enough to end such practices.

As we work toward prevention and focus on sustenance, we offer the best possible care to those on whom cancer has befallen. Cancer patients are the ones who warn us of the escalating crisis of imbalance in the world. We invite them to tell us what they are experiencing and thinking. We care for them holistically, involve them at every step of decision-making and communicate with them in clear and accessible language(s). Their economic, emotional, spiritual, and physical needs are paramount. Access is universal. Cost is never a barrier to early detection, treatment, and recovery.

There is excellent communication and collaboration among those with expertise and skills to offer. As we strive for the best possible outcome for cancer patients, there are no longer barriers separating research and practice, isolating specializations within the medical community, or impeding the integration of mainstream and complementary oncology. A holistic approach addressing the individual needs of each patient is timely, well-coordinated, integrative, and patient-centered.

There are now solid bridges in place between complementary and mainstream cancer care. Natural therapies proven to strengthen the immune system and fight cancer are funded by public health care and are administered by naturopathic oncologists working alongside medical oncologists and surgeons. The integrated model of care has definitively been shown to produce better outcomes at lower cost.

We support academic, health care, and other public institutions to educate, organize, carry out research, and communicate the sustainability issues of the day. All levels of government cooperate to plan, finance, and create accessible community-based support services and build awareness of the value of a healthier environment. New possibilities continually emerge as we work together to bring about the dream of a more balanced world.

Cancer is one of the most significant scourges of our times. There is too much loss, hardship, and suffering. A world where the causes and incidence of cancer are dramatically reduced and where patients receive optimal care will be a better world for all of us and for our children and grandchildren. The struggle is long, but hope is longer. My healers and my own struggle have taught me that a better world is possible.

Acknowledgments

I want to express my gratitude to the many wonderful people who traveled with me. From the bottom of my heart, I thank my oncologists Dr. Shailendra Verma and Dr. Joanne Meng, my surgeon Dr. Angel Arnaout, my naturopathic oncologist Dr. Leesa Kirchner, and my life coach Joyce Hardman. This "dream team" of healers used every conceivable strategy to fight my cancer, boost my immune system, and prevent a recurrence while tending to my body, soul, and spirit. Thanks too to my other health care providers Dr. Gerd Schneider, Dr. Mark de Gruchy and Amber McPhail and to dedicated staffers at the Women's Breast Health Centre at the Ottawa Hospital: Sandra Lowry, Linda Corsini, and Jennifer Smylie.

My heartfelt appreciation to all those who read my Healing Journey letters, who told me how the letters had touched their lives and urged me to keep on writing. And to Margie Wolfe of Second Story Press who saw possibilities in my letters during the dark days of treatment. She encouraged me to think about writing this book when

I didn't know if I'd make it and to carry on after I came out the other side. As the writing progressed, Kae McColl, James Loney, Larry Katz, Helen Levine, Fern Valin, Karen Levine, Kathryn Morrison and Dugald Seely offered invaluable input. Judy Field put in countless hours generously transcribing my interviews with the healers. Editor Sarah Swartz gave shape and structure to the manuscript in ways that eluded me until it landed in her hands, and editors Ruth Chernia and Carolyn Jackson helped polish it to completion. I am also grateful for the support of the Ontario Arts Council.

I couldn't have made it through treatment or the writing of this book without my women friends from near and far who were there in countless ways: commiserating, nurturing, strategizing, walking, cooking, driving, knitting, writing, meditating, and hanging out with me. Special thanks to the enthusiastic Supper Sister and Rad Rider teams brilliantly organized by Debbie Rubin and Denise Bisson. My survivor sisters Cathy Remus, Louise Vaillancourt, and Teresa Healy supported me with wisdom and love. Breast Friends, my support group, wholeheartedly believed in this book. I was inspired by the memory of Martha Segal.

My mother, Helen Zivian Levine, always encouraged me to write. She has been my loyal companion and booster through cancer and beyond, a wise woman who is loving, spirited, and insightful as she approaches 90. My father, Gil Levine, who died of acute leukemia soon after I started chemo, continues to sustain me in spirit. My best-ever sister Karen was with me every step of the way, watching the world with our special glasses and spending every post-chemo week-end with me.

The kids, Rachel, Daniel, and Eric, each embraced and supported me in their own way. My husband, Larry Katz, was at my side throughout this odyssey. As my staunch soul mate and lover, he was a shrewd strategist and tireless first mate as we strove to navigate the uncharted waters of the cancer care system. I am ever grateful for his constant love, for the supportive but critical eye he brought to my writing, and for his blessing to include some of the tough stuff in *But Hope is Longer.*

About the Author

TAMARA LEVINE is a long-time adult educator and literacy activist. She pioneered workplace literacy and clear language initiatives across Canada with the Ontario Federation of Labour and the Canadian Labour Congress. Following breast cancer treatment and recovery, she retired from her job in labor education in 2011. She lives in Ottawa with her family where she writes, sings, walks, and swims with the loons.

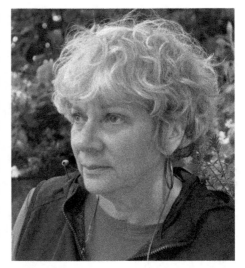

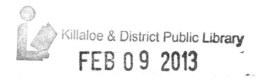